A KEATS GOOD HERB GUIDE

21



# HERBS FOR THE URINARY TRACT

*Herbal relief for kidney stones, bladder infections and other problems of the urinary tract.*

Michael Moore

Keats Publishing, Inc. New Canaan, Connecticut

*Herbs for the Urinary Tract* is not intended as medical advice. Its intent is solely informational and educational. Please consult a health professional should the need for one be indicated.

HERBS FOR THE URINARY TRACT



Library of Congress Cataloging-in-Publication Data

Moore, Michael, 1941–
Herbs for the urinary tract : herbal relief for kidney stones, bladder infections, and other problems of the urinary tract / Michael Moore.
p. cm.—(A Keats good herb guide)
Includes bibliographical references and index.
ISBN 0-87983-815-0
1. Urinary organs—Diseases—Alternative treatment. 2. Herbs—Therapeutic use. I. Title. II. Series.
RC900.5.M66 1998
616.6'06 dc21 98-15966
CIP

Printed in the United States of America

Keats Good Herb Guides are published by
Keats Publishing, Inc.
27 Pine Street (Box 876)
New Canaan, Connecticut 06840-0876
Website Address: www.keats.com

# *Contents*

CONTENTS

# *No More UTIs*

Self-limiting urinary tract or kidney problems will afflict nearly half the adult population at one time or another. The usual medical approach is antibiotics or anti-inflammatory drugs; they relieve the problem for a time, but the infection inevitably returns. The more frequent the recurrence, the more likely it is to eventually develop into a more serious disease state.

In this Good Herb Guide, herbalist Michael Moore examines the underlying causes of urinary tract disorders and shows how they can be managed with prevention, proper diet and the judicious use of some simple and safe herbs.

# *The author*

Michael Moore, considered the "Godfather of contemporary American herbalism," has been a professional herbalist for over 30 years. He has trained nearly a generation of herbalists through his school, the Southwest School of Botanical Medicine, and has written such books as *Medicinal Plants of the Mountain West, Medicinal Plants of the Desert and Canyon West, Medicinal Plants of the Pacific West* and *Los Remedios: Traditional Herbal Remedies of the Southwest.*

# *Introduction*

Probably half of us at some point in our lives will experience self-limiting urinary tract or kidney problems. Some of us will see a physician and take medication (with the problem usually recurring later), and others will suffer in silence and wait for the problem to simply go away.

Although medical care may be appropriate, frequently the medications taken will either suppress inflammation or simply kill microorganisms—in neither case is the underlying imbalance treated.

Those who binge on sugar consistently alter their urinary mucosa, creating a surface that bacteria can adhere to, and will often have recurrent urinary tract infections (UTIs) no matter how often they take antibiotics or how stoically they endure an infection that will eventually go away of its own accord, at least temporarily. The person with kidney stones who makes no change in diet or habits or stress is likely to have more stones.

The fact is, the more frequent the condition, the more likely it is to "ripen" into a more serious and organic disease state.

Most urinary tract problems can be managed by prevention, a little dietary discipline and the judicious use of some simple and safe herbs. In this book I intend to explain what goes on, what gets out of balance, and what you can do to prevent or treat these problems, using herbs and self-awareness.

# *Understanding Our Bodies*

## Living in the Ocean

Life as we know it evolved from single-celled organisms living within the sea and maintaining a dynamic balance between externally high levels of sodium and internally high levels of potassium. These life forms, then as now, pulled potassium into themselves while excreting excess sodium back out into the Mother Ocean . . . against the grain, as it were.

This artifact of holding high levels of internal potassium and low levels of internal sodium, while living in a milieu of high sodium and low potassium, creates immense stress on both sides of the cell's envelope, the membrane. The cell must expend energy (calories) to maintain this intentional imbalance between the internal media and the external media. Someone once said that life exists in response to irritation and stress. This electrolyte imbalance is, in fact, the very stress that enables living cells to absorb nutrients. They excrete waste products by using this membrane imbalance to transport in both directions across the celllular membrane—an energy fulcrum.

As long as a cell is alive, it maintains this imbalance. When it dies, sodium comes rushing in, and potassium is lost. The health of a cell can be partially defined by its efficiency in hoarding potassium while resisting and manipulating the greater sodium found in its external environment, the primordial and mythic Mother Ocean.

Take that cell and configure it into a colony of many similar cells—a simple multicellular organism such as a sponge—and each cell must stay in intimate contact with the surrounding ocean in order to maintain this electrolyte stress and health. With a multicellular organism that has several distinct layers of specialized cells, it becomes necessary to pump Mother Ocean through the organism so that the cells that lay within the mesodermal layer get their fair share of manipulatable sodium-potassium imbalance. They too, must absorb and excrete, no matter how buried they are in the sea slug or fish.

No matter how complex the animal or plant in this ocean, each cell must have access to a bath of sodium-rich and potassium-poor sea water . . . either directly or through the carefully maintained substitute of a closed-system imitation of the surf, a circulatory system that diffuses sea water through and over deeply buried masses of specialized cells.

In even the largest organism, each cell maintains the primordial necessity of being bathed in excess sodium while hoarding internally an excess of potassium and using its membrane to manipulate absorption and excretion—to, in effect, maintain itself as if it were a single cell floating in salty water.

This seemingly labored method of treating each cell as if it lived autonomously is all fine and dandy when you are living right in the middle of that very same salty water: the ocean. A method as inefficient as the workings of the internal combustion engine in an automobile, its how things are done, how they have always been done. It does, after all, work.

## Living on the Land

When life forms first started to creep onto dry land (400 to 500 million years ago, give or take an eon), they took with them this tried-and-true method of sodium and potassium stress manipulation—except there was no Mother Ocean surrounding them. Plants and animals further elaborated the concept of a closed circulatory system to the point that, by closing off their surfaces to the air and pumping a recreation of sea water through their bodies, they could convince their cells that they still lived in the ocean. Plants and animals on the land had to, in effect, start carrying bags of synthetic sea water inside them . . . a salty water bringing food to cells and taking waste products from them, a functional substitute for the washing waters of the sea.

This brought up a problem, particularly as plants and animals moved further away from coastal regions: how to get enough sodium to maintain the internal "sea water" that must, by necessity, be rich in sodium and poor in potassium.

In the ocean, larger animals had to gather sodium from their cells and excrete it out into the water. On the land, plants and especially animals had to gather sodium from their surroundings and hoard it internally. This, in order to keep that well-oiled sodium-potassium imbalance, an imbalance easy to maintain in the ocean, far more complex on dry land. Land animals evolved mechanisms that had to become increasingly efficient at keeping that circulating "ocean" within a very narrow range of salinity, diffusing free gases through it by way of lungs and gathering the dissolved waste products drawn off from the cells into concentrated fluids held in an organ that could then excrete them from the whole colony of cells.

How does this relate to urinary tract problems?

- We carry our ocean within us as lymph and blood.
- We diffuse gases through lymph and blood by respiring with our lungs.
- We maintain the salinity and volume of our internal "ocean" with our kidneys.
- We concentrate a small amount of the processed

"ocean" as urine and carry waste products from the blood onto the urine, and thence into the bladder, where we hold it until it reaches sufficient volume to excrete.

- The kidneys maintain the ocean and hold back almost everything suspended in that "ocean." Urine is a side effect of what the kidneys do and intimately reflects the ongoing nature of ocean/lymph/blood/lung chemistry and the kidneys' control of those fluids.
- Most urinary tract problems occur because there is an ongoing imbalance in "ocean" chemistry, with major shifts in the concentration, salinity or acid/alkaline balance of urine.
- Although it is usually possible, after the fact, to inhibit a UTI infection or soothe irritated and painful membranes with herbs, the best results occur by also rectifying the underlying cause of metabolic stress that changes the quality of the ocean and therefore alters both the function of the kidneys and the nature of urine.

The patterns of imbalances for which herbal preventives and herbal treatments work best are those induced by stress and diet. These usually occur together, since stress itself compounds the effects of a poor diet, and faulty diet induces further stress.

Virtually every urinary tract problem starts from metabolic imbalances. At every stage it is important to examine personal patterns of stress and, besides using herbs to treat symptoms, use a tonic or make the appropriate changes in diet to alleviate the conditions underlying the UTI.

Chances are, if you have had a urinary tract problem, you will have another under similar conditions. Therefore, learning how to balance yourself is as important as learning how to treat yourself.

Before considering these aspects, we'll take a brief look at the mechanics of the urinary tract and then briefly consider the broad patterns of stress and how they affect the urinary tract.

# The Kidneys

The kidneys take arterial blood from the renal arteries and squeeze it through half-a-million little filter tubes (the nephrons) which separate the blood into thick protein sludge and watery serum. The serum passes lymph-like through the tubes, allowing all the important constituents to be absorbed back into the sludge until the exiting blood is restored and cleaned. A minute amount of fluid (containing waste solutes and acids) is passed out into the kidney pelvis and ureters as urine. The result is that sodium or potassium is retained (under the influence of the adrenal cortex), water is retained or not (the pituitary) and the acid/alkaline balance is maintained. The overall control of acid and alkaline is the joint effort of the kidneys and lungs.

Further, the compensatory reactivity and constriction of blood vessels and the heart is potentiated by kidney proteins, which are acted on by the liver and activated in the tissues. The kidneys produce renin, which is manipulated further by the liver and liver-synthesized protein and becomes vasoconstricting, when needed, in blood vessels. This allows blood to flow to the brain when we stand, to back off when we sit, etc. Basically, the kidneys' primary function is to control blood volume, quality and dispersal, with urine production simply a means to this end. The kidneys are organs that hold in far more than they let out.

## Deficiency Symptoms

Most usually the result of adrenalin ("flight-or-fight") stress, symptoms include frequent, dilute and pale urination (often at night), flushing, thirst and the tendency to low blood pressure. Orthostatic hypotension is common—when standing up the blood stays somewhere around the solar plexus, gradually surging up to the brain. If the kidneys and arteries fail to compensate fast enough, the kidney-deficient person compensates by sitting down dizzily or, if this fails, by fainting.

There is a tendency to react poorly to sudden changes in temperature and humidity, with frequent short-term water retention and headaches. Common stresses to fluid and osmosis homeostasis, such as PMS, changes in barometric pressure, high altitudes, the last trimester of pregnancy, steroid drugs and high salt intake produce exaggerated symptoms in the kidney-deficient person.

The urine more easily becomes neutral or alkaline, easily shifting from its normal acidity with even moderate alterations in diet.

## Kidney Deficiency Tonics

These either strengthen or stimulate kidney nephrons, improve renal blood supply that is diminished in adrenalin stress and improve hormonal stimulation.

- **Dong quai** (cured *Angelica sinensis*)
- **Shepherd's purse** (*Capsella bursa-pastoris*)
- **Horsetail** (*Equisetum arvense* and others)
- **Licorice root** (*Glycyrrhiza glabra* and others)
- **Ginseng** (all: *Panax, Eleutherococcus,* etc.)
- **Huckleberry or blueberry** (*Vaccinium spp.*)

With kidney deficiency and increased volume of urine,

there is less fluid surplus for the skin, intestines and lungs. Since there is only a finite volume of saline fluid (Mother Ocean) that the body is willing to excrete outwards, if any one surface consistently hypersecretes, the other surfaces have less water potential. This is easily observed in someone who is working hard and sweating profusely: urine will often be concentrated, even scalding, and constipation frequently follows. Excessive skin fluids are being thrown out and the body hoards other fluids to compensate. With the excessive urination of kidney deficiency, dry skin and constipation often follow, and even the bronchial membranes can become dry.

Licorice root shifts fluids away from the kidneys and increases the fluid investment in the other membranes.

Dong quai and the ginsengs all moderately increase anabolic metabolism and the utilization of aldosterone while increasing protein metabolism and blood supply to the kidneys. Shepherd's purse and huckleberry or blueberry are astringent to the nephrons, and horsetail helps to strengthen their connective tissues.

**Kidney Deficiency Tincture**

| | |
|---|---|
| Licorice root tincture | 2 parts |
| Shepherd's purse tincture | 2 parts |
| Siberian ginseng tincture | 2 parts |
| Dong quai tincture | 1 part |

Combine and take 60 drops (2 squirts) 3X a day in a bit of warm water.

## KIDNEY DEFICIENCY NERVINES

If you are prone to chronic flight-or-fight adrenaline stress, with easy agitation, constipation and allergies (along with kidney deficiency) you might try Pulsatilla tincture (3–5 drops when agitated), homeopathic *Pulsatilla* 6x or 12x, St. John's wort, blue vervain tea (2–4 ounces of a standard infusion), or, my favorite, 3–5 drops of fresh lobelia tincture. These are all meant to soothe, not sedate.

**Dietary changes.** Choose foods with a slower rate of sugar metabolism (see Glycemic Index, page 84) and add some type of slowly digested food (such as butter or olive oil) to any consumption of high-index foods (such as carrots or potatoes). Binging on candy or other quick-fuel foods will always jolt brain, liver, digestive and kidney metabolism in a negative way. Further, induced vomiting or the use of cathartics (bolemic mechanisms) usually supports this pattern of addictive eating. Adding some low glycemic index foods will gradually wean the liver away from turning everything you eat directly into fuel.

Bear in mind that the glycemic index of a food often has little bearing on its basic nutritional value; it simply indicates just how quickly the food alters the blood sugar levels, both up or down. Organic carrot juice is a good source of nutrients but a poor food for stabilizing blood sugar and kidney-deficiency problems. Peanut butter is very easy on the glycemic/kidney axis, but very high in fat. Balance is the key.

Taking 20 to 30 drops of Oregon grape (*Mahonia spp.*) tincture before each meal often helps digestive and liver functions keep up with a gradual change in diet.

Remember that adrenalin stress excessively alters a variety of metabolic pathways. If you consider yourself an adrenalin-stressed person with kidney deficiency, you probably are dealing with some urinary tract problems. That means you probably inherited a less-than-ideal urinary tract. When under stress others may show problems in digestion, allergies, blood sugar stability or blood pressure. You are likely to experience urinary track stress. You need to lessen your stress profile in order to get over recurrent kidney or bladder problems. It isn't enough to patch things up every time they hurt; you must start preventing the problem.

## EXCESS SYMPTOMS

Kidney excess symptoms include sodium and water retention; essential hypertension (from increased blood volume); concentrated acidic urine; warm, moist skin (under any circumstance) and orthostatic hypertension (you stand up quickly and it feels as if blood is trying to pound out through your ears and crown chakra). A person with these symptoms usually craves proteins and fats, sweats easily, and, under stress, relies not on quick adrenaline-type responses but instead tends to increase bulk, store fuel for the winter and metabolically dig in for the long haul. Think mesomorph and meaty.

Remember that, by and large, the kidneys simply do what is necessary to compensate for necessary or unnecessary shifts in general metabolism. Most imbalances of kidney function arise from physical and emotional stress. Much of this is habitual and, to some degree, avoidable.

## KIDNEY EXCESS TONICS

These work in two possible ways. (1) Metabolic coolers: relax the limbic system and the hypothalamus and decrease kidney reabsorption of sodium, therefore increasing the volume of the urine (since water follows sodium); or (2) Diuretic coolers: decrease water reabsorption by altering osmosis in the nephrons, with sodium following.

Food is very important here; decrease protein in the diet and increase foods high in electrolytes and minerals.

**Metabolic Coolers**

- **Pleurisy root** (*Asclepias tuberosa*)

- **Blue flag** (*Iris versicolor* or *I. missouriensis*)

**Diuretic Coolers**

- **Burdock** (*Arctium lappa* or *A. minus*)
- **Shepherd's purse** (*Capsella bursa-pastoris*)
- **Canadian fleabane** (*Conyza [Erigeron] canadense*)
- **Horsetail** (*Equisetum arvense* and others)
- **Dandelion** (*Taraxacum spp.*)

**Kidney Excess Formula**

| | |
|---|---|
| Burdock root | 2 parts |
| Dandelion root | 2 parts |
| Pleurisy root | 1 part |
| Siberian ginseng | 1 part |

Combine the four herbs (based on weight), boil ½ ounce of the formula in a pint of water (a strong decoction), and drink ⅓ of the strained tea in three portions during the day.

# *Lower Urinary Tract*

Urine collects slowly from the inner surface of each of the kidneys and drips into the funnel-like renal pelvis. When enough urine has gathered, a contraction squeezes it down into the ureter, and, from this point, as in all muscular ducts of the body, the small bolus of urine is milked down to the bladder. There may be several such urine masses descending towards the bladder at any one time.

The ureters have two methods of muscle activity. One, under sympathetic adrenergic control, constricts band-like and blocks urine passage. The other muscular urges are downward contractions under the stimulus of parasympathetic cholinergic nerves. As is so frequent in our bodies, the passage is orderly *because* it entails the cooperation of opposing forces. There must be enough urine and muscular energy to overcome the constricting muscles and force a bolus of urine downwards. This is the same action as that which allows food to pass downwards through the gut and bile through the biliary apparatus. Balance is the result of opposing energies.

There must be additional muscular contractions to squirt the bolus into the bladder, since both the two entrances and the exit of the bladder are under constricting sympathetic adrenergic control. So is the muscular basement of the bladder to which they are attached, the trigone muscle. The bladder expands as the urine collects, and this is controlled by the detrusor muscles—under parasympathetic nerve stimulus—a similar balance between constriction and expansion as is found in the ureters.

When enough urine has collected, the trigone and its sphincters relax, the detrusor contracts outwards, voluntary relaxation (from the brain and spinal cord) occurs and we urinate. Sounds complicated—no wonder it took us a year or two (or three) to learn to do all this!

Lower urinary tract stress occurs from the same factor as causes kidney deficiency: adrenaline stress.

Remember that the main function of the kidneys is to hold in the Mother Ocean. Adrenalin stress and the common dietary shifts it induces tend to lessen the kidneys' abilities to do this.

The main function of the lower urinary tract is to gather the urine produced during this process by the kidneys and collect it for eventual evacuation. Adrenalin stress *constricts* the passage of urine and inhibits the parasympathetic milking of the ureters and the expelling of the detrusor.

As in defecation, urination is inhibited by adrenaline excess. During the usual pattern of daytime adrenalin stress, there is a certain grim harmony; the kidneys produce less urine, and the lower urinary tract holds on to it longer. They had *all* better relax by evening. The kidneys, in rebound, will produce more urine, and the lower urinary tract should *also* be relaxed and pass urine more easily.

If all things are not equal, there can be a tendency for incomplete bladder evacuation (from residual constriction) or the urge to frequent, low-volume urination, which is stressful on the urethra and weakening to the detrusor muscle, as it is seldom allowed to expand adequately. Without regular expansion and contraction, it can actually shrink—as the stomach can when little food is eaten for an extended period.

The same tonic herbs and dietary changes should be used for lower urinary tract stress as for kidney deficiency (see above).

# *Cystitis and Urethritis*

## Preventing UTIs

In the healthy individual, a number of factors keep the lower urinary tract in balance.

For starters, as in all entrances into the body, there is a healthy community of native flora in the urethra. These are tolerated and even encouraged by the body, and our immunity is careful not to attack them. They flourish and dominate when the local environment is stable and consistent. Because they dominate and are amicable to that environment, other organisms cannot compete and seldom take hold.

This is also true in the colon, where good digestive functions nurture similar beneficial flora and poor digestion changes the colon environment and the balance and type of intestinal flora . . . often with low-level inflammation resulting.

Change the environment in the mouth and the normal flora becomes abnormal; the gums become puffy and the tongue becomes coated. Changes in environment also affect the vagina, the upper bronchial membranes, the ears, and the skin.

In a healthy urethra, the dominant bacteria are the *Lactobacillus* group, and in women the dominant healthy organisms of the vagina are also *Lactobacilli*. They thrive well in the acidity of the lower urinary tract and the vagina.

Further, the acid wastes of the urine—urea, uric acid and other organic acids—help to maintain the osmolality or electrical charge of the whole tract, especially the repelling charges on the surface membranes of the mucosa. This helps to keep the surface clean and resistant to any but small amounts of friendly organisms.

Then there are the simple mechanics of bacterial infections . . . they can't swim *upstream* when there is regular evacuation of normal urine going *downstream*. They can move upstream, however, when there are long periods of adrenalin stress with infrequent urination followed by renal overcompensation with watery urine having a low acidity and charge or when there is incomplete evacuation of the bladder.

In addition, the bladder has several defense mechanisms of its own to clear out bacteria, including the release of antibodies into the urine and the production of specialized mucus starches that clump up bacteria, block their attachment and clear them out of the bladder through the urine. In men, prostate secretions are further inhibitors of infection.

In general then, the free flow of acidic urine, full urine volume, complete emptying of the bladder and healthy immune functions are the body's best antibacterial defenses.

## What Causes UTIs

Bladder infections in women are surprisingly common. Twenty-one percent of all women have some urinary tract discomfort at least once a year, 37.5 percent of women with no previous urinary tract infection will have an episode within ten years and up to 4 percent of apparently healthy women have elevated levels of abnormal bacteria in their urine, presumably from an asymptomatic infection.

Further, women with a history of recurrent UTIs will usually have an episode at least once every year. Recurrent bladder infections can be a significant problem for some women . . . 55 percent will eventually involve the kidneys, since the same conditions that allow reoccurring infections can allow the infection to ascend up the urinary tract. Recurrent kidney infections can cause progressive damage resulting in scarring and, for a few, kidney failure. By the time the kidneys are involved, herbs and natural approaches are often inadequate, since such infections, more dangerous and profound, usually need medical intervention.

Herbs are most effective in the lower urinary tract and support the lessening of metabolic stress.

Urinary tract infections in males are much less common and usually indicate an anatomical abnormality, a sexually transmitted disease or a prostate infection. Urinary tract infections are rare in boys (0.05 percent) while only 2 percent of girls have excessive bacteria in their urine. Part of this is because growing children, with a rapid rate of growth and metabolic heat tend to have strongly acidic urine and maintain a strong charge in both the urine *and* the urinary tract mucosa. Few bacteria can thrive under these circumstances.

Factors that increase the risk for UTIs are pregnancy (twice as frequent), sexual intercourse (nuns, as an example, have only 10 percent as many), trauma and irritation (such as a 1,000-mile trek in a subcompact car with only coffee breaks), anal intercourse and any structural blockages, such as urethral scar tissue and BPH (benign prostatic hyperplasia).

A number of other factors can affect an individual's predisposition to UTI. As mentioned, women are more susceptible than men since the urethra is shorter and more easily in contact with colon flora. Further, some women are naturally more disposed to recurrent infection, presumably the result of genetic factors that allow the mucous membranes to be more receptive to bacterial attachment.

Age in another factor, with between 10–20 percent of

elderly people experiencing UTIs. Similarly, folks with diabetes may have three times as many infections.

Hospital catheterization and the use of a diaphragm with spermicides also increase the frequency of infections.

During the development of urinary tract infections, a key factor is that infectious bacteria develop the ability to adhere to the mucous membranes of the urethra and bladder, thereby avoiding the normal resistance that combines to flush them out in the urine.

And finally, the colon bacteria that cause most UTIs (*E. coli* alone is found as the dominant organism 90 percent of the time) bind to carbohydrate or sugar residues on the surface of the lower urinary tract mucosa. It isn't only diabetes that can raise the level of sugar in the urine; simple bingeing on sweets can result in a short-term flushing of urinary sugar as well. Many a urinary tract infection follows the day after a late-night binge on Oreo cookies.

It is unfortunate that the primary bacterial causes of UTIs are endemic organisms. Like the *lactobacilli* in the vagina and urethra, *E. coli* are a necessary part of stable flora in the colon. It's just that, when they cause an infection in the urinary tract, there are no antibodies made to resist them and all the tissues there can do is respond to their presence with healing (and painful) inflammation. There can be no specific bacterial resistance formed to a normally "friendly" bug . . . even if it shows up in the wrong place. One of the flaws in dosing oneself with urinary antibiotics for such a reoccurring infection is that it strips away all the friendly bacteria, and the *E. coli* are just sitting there an inch or so away, a constant potential for reinfection. Moreover, antibiotics make no change in the weakened ecology of the urethra and bladder, fail to strengthen native urinary tract resistance and have no effect on the metabolic and habit factors that allow infections to begin with.

It has been my observation over the years that women with reoccurring UTIs also suffer a high rate of vaginal infections . . . either Candida or the more complex syndrome of bacterial vaginosis. All three conditions share a local deficiency of *lactobacillus* bacteria, and all can be aggravated by the frequent shifts in blood sugar that result from both bingeing and adrenalin stress, with infectious bacteria able to initiate membrane attachment because of abnormal sugar residues on the mucosa.

## Prevention Philosophy

In terms of prevention it is good, for starters, to examine your image of yourself as a viable and robust organism. We all have orifices where things go in and things go out. It's normal. These openings are populated with a fierce variety of organisms. They reflect the secretions, excretions and environments of those openings. They *belong* there and need to be there. We are, in a manner of perception, walking colonies of friendly organisms. We cannot and should not be clean, slick and sterile; we must, however be in balance. If we are in balance, so are our friendly organisms. They act as a living shield against outside organisms that can cause infection.

A consistent environment and lifestyle, coupled with reasonably good health, allow every surface of our body to harbor complex mixtures of microorganisms—those specifically evolved to live on our secretions and excretions and whose health and dominance depends intimately on our maintaining a consistent internal metabolism so that what comes off our body maintains a consistent culturing medium.

This may seem like a peculiar vision of ourselves, given our culture's obsession with cleansing, cleaning, washing, brushing, spraying, douching and disinfecting all parts of the body as if we were under constant bombardment by noxious evils. We are. Normal, healthy, "clean" people like you and me have mites living on their skin, in their eyelash follicles, in their hair and bacteria and fungi everywhere else. We are not sterile; rather we are in balance, first within, then without.

True, the urethra is a private concern, found in a private place and heavily weighted with sexual and excretory tension. Nonetheless, cystitis, like hemorrhoids, reminds us firmly and painfully of some of our more homely physical attributes. It might not hurt, therefore, to start off by visualizing the simple imperatives.

We urinate fluids that aid in metabolic balance through a surface orifice in close proximity to another excretory orifice. Good urine maintains normal flora and repels flora from the *other* orifice. Health is not being "clean and spotless" (we are not, after all, surgical devices). Health is balance. Prevention of cystitis needs to begin by finding out what agents are preventing balance.

In general, it is always preferable to *stop* doing something that may aggravate a condition such as cystitis (and see if it helps) rather than to journey blindly through a series of therapeutic approaches. If you are *doing* things that help sustain a discomfort, it is unlikely that treating it therapeutically, without lifestyle changes, will have anything more than short-term benefit—just as the asthmatic will need stronger and more invasive treatment as long as he continues to smoke or live in a polluted environment. Nearly all of us have been brainwashed into believing that the answer to a problem is best dealt with by going out and getting some new stuff. One rarely steps back and attempts self-evaluation to try and figure out what we are going that may be contributing to physical problems. We, as a society, tend to presume that we need to do some *more* stuff, rather than *less* stuff; we are consummate consumers.

What follows are some factors to consider that may be pertinent to one person and not to another. Each factor is a potential aggravation to cystitis that should be considered as just that: *potential.*

A person with frequent bladder infections may be eating

sugar six times a day (and altering the surface of the bladder mucosa), be under constant adrenalin stress, thus slowing kidney function and urine transport, or wearing tight pants with synthetic-fabric underwear (and holding secretions, sweat and heat tightly to one body area). These are ongoing habits that perpetuate 24-hour-a-day stress on the urethra and bladder. You cannot expect to drink herbal tea for three days twice a year and undo all the imbalances that your lifestyle itself has wrought.

If you wish to use herbs (less toxic and invasive measures that are under your own control), then you must take some preventive and tonic steps as well. Herbal approaches are not strong enough to suppress pathologies or supplant poor defenses; their relative "weakness" is their grace. If you find that sugar is an underpinning to your cystitis, and you can't cut down consumption, then you can expect no more than palliative relief from taking herbs.

## Mechanical Causes of Cystitis

**Tampons:** External napkins may be preferable.

**Vaginal sponges:** A nice idea, but they can often end up harboring the very bacteria that sustain an infection (and beware of sneezing!)

**Clothing:** Synthetic fabrics, especially polyester, will usually aggravate. Stick with cotton.

**Contraceptives:** Spermicidal gels, generic condoms, those bizarre, fluorescent, "articulated" penile covers favored by neoadolescent males and the various contraceptive vaginal jams and jellies can all variously aggravate concurrent cystitis/vaginitis. Make sure that a diaphragm fits properly; it can cause abrasions on insertion or extraction if it fits poorly. For women still using IUDs, beware. They can be a major factor in contributing to cystitis. For males, friction from a poorly fitted diaphragm and some of the older

IUDs can set up a cycle of urethral irritation, as can some spermicidal gels.

**Soap and cosmetics:** Strong antimicrobial soaps like Safeguard may alter (sometimes to the worse) surface flora. Scented, flavored or colored vaginal or anal lubricants offer up a variety of possible allergens or irritants. Some scented bath oils, surfactants and salts may also irritate the urethra and labia, as can use of those scented "feminine" sprays, douches and such. Even excess douching with more staid agents can contribute to the disruption of the normal flora.

## Sexual Activities

**Vaginal intercourse:** Like it or not, the more frequent, the more cystitis. The more partners, the more cystitis. "Honeymoon cystitis" is even worse . . . frequent intercourse with a new partner. Women under 20 years of age bear the greatest risk, since the hormonal yo-yos of adolescence can contribute to a chronic imbalance of vaginal pH and major shifts in native flora, both compromising resistance.

**Anal intercourse:** A sure way to aggravate or even initiate cystitis in males—use a condom. If vaginal intercourse follows, at the very least change condoms—anything else puts your partner at risk for cystitis. If you are a male with recurring cystitis, anal intercourse is generally the *last* thing you should be doing. Find inventive alternatives.

**Oral sex:** Mouth flora is *very* changeable and infectious bacteria can be passed back and forth this way. If you are trying to deal with frequent urethritis and cystitis, oral sex may be contributing.

**Oral contraceptives and pregnancy:** I realize this is a peculiar juxtaposition of terms, but, to a degree, the first mimics the second, and membrane resistance is lower in both cases.

**Sexual abuse sequelae:** Men and especially women with a history of overt sexual abuse or general physical abuse have consistently greater incidence of cystitis later in life. The explanations are many, varied and conflicting, and certainly beyond the scope of herb use and this little book. From whatever subtle and very human mechanisms, you should at the least consider this as a deep undercurrent to be dealt with however you must. Acknowledging such a cause and honoring its effects on you may help you avoid endless pursuit of externalized treatment.

## TREATMENT OF UTIs

### Diet

Obviously, in light of the effects of refined and unrefined sugar on the urinary tract mucosa, reduce as much as possible the consumption of any sweets. This includes such "correct" foods as sweet vegetables and fruits, honey and those genially fraudulent "health" bars. Avoid processed foods, snack foods, and those pseudoedibles with four or five lines of constituents on the package.

- Avoid artificially sweetened foods. Except for licorice and Stevia, all the synthetic sweets are hard on the kidneys and urinary tract.
- Avoid foods that contain "FD&C" coloring agents, although plant pigments derived from annatto, turmeric and chlorophyll are fine.
- It is generally beneficial to try to acidify the urine, although this is easier said than done. It may be simpler to decrease foods that are alkaline-forming such as milk, citrus juices and sodas.

- Avoid sour foods, spices, citrus fruits, tomatoes, alcohol, caffeine and other central nervous system stimulants.
- Eliminate overt bladder irritants, which may increase your discomfort, such as coffee, black tea and alcohol (particularly wine). Chocolate can also have a negative effect in some cases.
- The following foods can also irritate an existing UTI: Apples, grapes, canned figs, raisins, peaches, pineapple, cantaloupe, citrus fruits, bananas, guavas, nectarines, avocados, chicken liver, brewer's yeast, soy sauce, fava beans, corned beef, nuts, chocolate, pickled herring, beer (especially dark), wine (especially red), vinegar, mayonnaise and fermented or cultured dairy products such as sour cream, yogurt and hard cheeses. After the UTI has passed, resume eating yogurt for its beneficial lactobacillus.
- Drink large amounts of water—eight ounces an hour. It will help flush the bacteria out of your system and will often reduce pain on urination.
- While you are treating a UTI, eat a light diet consisting of grains, some vegetables and cranberry or blueberry juices.

## Supplements, Nutritional and Otherwise

- Vitamin C, either in tablet or powder, can irritate the bladder, and is best taken in a buffered form, such as calcium ascorbate.
- Avoid vitamins containing aspartate, as it is a bladder irritant.

- **Do take:**
  Vitamin E—400 to 600 IU/day
  Vitamin B6—300 mg/day
- Potassium citrate and/or sodium citrate have long been employed in the treatment of lower urinary tract infections. Although they clearly alkalize the urine, not every-

thing pertaining to UTIs can be reduced simply to a matter of pH. There are some clinical studies to support this practice.

In a study reported in Pizzorno and Murray's *Textbook of Natural Medicine,* women presenting with symptoms of a urinary tract infection were given a 4 g dose of sodium citrate every 8 hours for 48 hours. Of the 64 women evaluated, 80 percent had relief of symptoms, 12 percent had deterioration of symptoms, and 91.8 percent of the women rated the treatment as acceptable.

- One teaspoon of baking soda in one-half cup of water once or twice a day will also alkalinize the urine.

**What about Cranberry juice?**

The effect of cranberry juice on urinary tract infections has been investigated sporadically for the past 35 years, with increasing evidence that it can and should be used as an aid in the prevention of the more common alkaline-urine UTIs.

The earliest investigations into the mode of action of cranberry juice focused on its effects on the acidity of the urine and increased concentration of hippuric acid in the urine. However, it was found that the increase in acidity was in fact minor, with little apparent effect on infection. In addition, although hippuric acid is known to possess bacteriostatic properties, the levels in the urine are unimportant, except in helping to maintain that peculiar nitrogen acid charge of healthy urine that is so important in supporting the mucous membranes.

More recent studies have clearly shown that cranberry juice and cranberry juice with fructose can inhibit the adherence of *E.coli* to human urinary tract mucus cells. The next step was to identify the constituents of cranberry juice which contribute to the anti-adherence activity.

It has been found that the juice contains at least two adherence inhibitors; the first is low molecular weight. The low MW compound specifically inhibited the activity of a common strain of *E. coli* associated with UTIs. The low MW compound has been identified and constitutes the fructose component of the juice where it is believed to interfere with the mannose-specific lectin on the *E.coli* wall binding to the reception site on the epithelial cell surface.

Fructose itself had no inhibitory action on the other strain of *E. coli* with UTI implications; however, the high MW compound found in cranberry juice was found to profoundly inhibit them. Fructose-enriched cranberry juice therefore has the potential to inhibit the attachment of both types of *E. coli* which are most commonly associated with UTI.

***In vivo* studies with cranberry juice.** In the first major study of the use of cranberry juice in treating UTI, it was found that 32 patients out of 60 showed a positive clinical response, 12 were moderately improved and 16 showed no improvement.

Further studies found that between 12 and 30 ounces of raw unpasteurized cranberry juice daily was a good preventive treatment for many types of urinary tract infections. On further study, it was found that there was statistically significant anti-adherence activity in human urine from 1 to 3 hours after drinking a 25 percent dilution of fructose-enriched cranberry juice.

In order for bacteria to infect, they must first adhere to the mucosa. By interfering with adherence, cranberry juice greatly reduces the likelihood of infection and helps the body fight off infection. This is the most likely explanation of the positive effects of cranberry juice in bladder infections.

In studies, the anti-adherence compounds secreted in the urine were very similar to the original cranberry juice mix, indicating these factors moved easily from the digestive system, through the bloodstream and out into the urinary tract. Most *E. coli* strains implicated in UTIs utilize two types of adhering proteins, and for any agent to exert a positive effect, it should be against both types. Cranberry juice does this, and its constituents excreted in the urine *also* do this.

In fact, straight cranberry juice can cause 99 percent inhibition of attachment, and even a 1/100 dilution causes significant reduction.

It was found that the successful inhibition of attachment occurred in over 60 percent of *E. coli* strains isolated from urinary tract infections, although it was less effective on intestinal strains.

In one study of seven juices (cranberry, blueberry, grapefruit, quava, mango, orange, and pineapple) only cranberry and blueberry contained this inhibitor.[3] Blueberry juice is a suitable alternative to cranberry juice in bladder infections.

It must be pointed out that most cranberry juices on the market contain one-third cranberry juice mixed with water and sugar. Since sugar (sucrose) has a detrimental effect on the immune system, and, as mentioned before, can contribute to bacterial attachments on the mucosa, use of sweetened cranberry juice cannot be recommended. Fresh cranberry (sweetened with apple or grape juice) or blueberry juice is preferred. Cranberry extracts are also available commercially in pill form.

## Herbs

After modifying stresses by making lifestyle and diet changes and adding some tonic herbs, you need to decide whether to use a single herb for your cystitis (best for simple, uncomplicated, acute UTIs) or put together a formula (best for frequent or more chronic conditions).

If you wish to try a single herb, one of the antimicrobials is best (see page 28).

For a formula, it is usually best to use an herb from each of the following categories (see page 28–32):

1. Urinary antimicrobial
2, 3. Urinary demulcent, astringent or both
4. Diuretic
5, 6. Urinary analgesic, anti-inflammatory or both
7. Urinary antispasmodic (optional)

*A note on making your own formula:* Some herbs make fine teas, some herbs work best as tinctures, some as either. It may be easier to make *either* a tea or tincture formula. However, it is perfectly possible to put together a formula by making a tea of two herbs and adding the rest of the herbs as tinctures (or some variant thereof).

Finally, most formulas commercially available either focus on "fluid retention" or mindlessly combine urinary tract herbs together with little thought to the philosophy of treatment, just combining the herbs for UTIs listed in *Back to Eden* and thus adding yet another preparation to their product line. It is best to put together your own formula.

Most herbs for UTIs are readily available on the marketplace, but some of them may take a little work locating. Therefore, I suggest you make your own herbal preparation out of what's available to you where you live. I have listed a great number of herbs here, many with similar effects, so that it will be easy for you to assemble a formula at your local co-op, health food store or herb store.

Although many tea plants could be tinctured, I recommend tincturing only if some parts of the plant are insoluble in water, the herb is most active in the fresh state and needs to be preserved in that form, or if the herb is so potent that a few drops or a squirt supplies a physiologically active dosage.

For example, one could tincture alfalfa, but the effect of the alcohol would end up being greater than the constituents. You might need a tablespoon of alfalfa tincture to be effective—enough alcohol to get some of us tipsy.

In each section below, I have listed my favorite herbs first. These are generally those I know best; you may find another herb works just fine.

***1. Urinary Antimicrobials.*** These herbs are all related and contain similar constituents that are excreted in the urine and inhibit bacteria. They are generally most effective when the urine is alkaline. Those high in tannins are best used in short-term acute treatment. Those low in tannins can be used either short-term or in formulas.

*High in Tannins*

- **Uva Ursi** (*Arctostaphylos uva-ursi*), tea or tincture.
- **Manzanita** (*Arctostaphylos spp.*, bushes native to California and the Southwest), tea or tincture.

*Low in Tannins*

- **Pipsissewa** (*Chimaphila umbellata*), tea or tincture.
- **Huckleberry** or **blueberry** (*Vaccinium spp.*), tea.

*Aromatic Antimicrobials*

These are effective primarily because they contain essential oils or oleoresins that are excreted in the urine and variously inhibit organisms adhering to the mucosa or have involved the cell layers below. Some are rather safe for either short-term or formula use ("general use"); others are strong and potentially irritating to either the stomach, kidneys or the bladder mucosa itself ("industrial strength") and are best used in small quantities as part of a formula.

*General Use*

- **Yerba mansa** (*Anemopsis californica*), tea or tincture.
- **Cubeb berries** (*Piper cubeba*), tea or tincture.

- **Buchu** (*Agothasma* or *Barosma spp.*), tea or tincture.
- **Yerba santa** (*Eriodictyon californica* or *E. angustifolia*), tea or tincture.
- **Eucalyptus leaves** (*Eucalyptus globulus*), tea.
- **Grindelia** (*Grindelia spp.*), tea or tincture.
- **Juniper leaves** (*Juniperus spp.*), tea.

*Industrial Strength*

- **Juniper berries** (*Juniperus communis*), Tea or tincture (do not use oil of juniper).
- **Myrrh gum** or **Guggul** (*Commiphora spp.*), tincture.

*Anticandida-Antifungal*

These are herbs that inhibit candida in both the urinary tract and the vagina. All are safe for short-term or long-term use.

- **Fireweed** or **Great Willow Herb** (*Epilobium angustifolium*), tea.
- **Yerba mansa** (*Anemopsis californica*), tea or tincture.
- **Pau d'arco** (*Tabebuia spp.*), tea or capsule.

2. ***Urinary Astringents.*** These are herbs that either shrink swollen membranes, contract boggy membranes into a more resistant tone or diminish and stop hypersecretions and bleeding from membranes.

- **Shepherd's purse** (*Capsella bursa-pastoris*), tea or tincture (recently picked plant only).
- **Canadian fleabane** (*Conyza [Erigeron] canadense*), tea.
- **Yarrow** (*Achillea millefolium*), tea or tuncture.
- **Mormon tea** (*Ephedra viridis, E. nevadensis,* etc.), tea (not to be confused with *Ephedra sinica* or other Asian species sold as Ma Huang).
- **Rose buds** (*Rosa spp.*), tea.
- **Rosemary** (*Rosmarinus spp.*), tea.

- **Agrimony** (*Agrimonia spp.*), tea.
- **Ladies mantle** (*Alchemilla*), tea.
- **Cranesbill** or **Wild Geranium** (*Geranium spp.*), tea.

*3.* ***Urinary Demulcents.*** These contain specialized starches that, after being excreted in the urine, act as mucus analogues. They also stimulate increased protective mucus secretions.

- **Marshmallow** or **Hollyhock** (*Althea officinalis* or *A. rosea*), tea.
- **Corn silk** (*Zea Mays*), tea.

*4.* ***Diuretics.*** These act to increase the volume of urine, usually without increasing solids. Although there are herbs that stimulate urine production by increasing blood flow to the kidneys, these usually have the potential to irritate the kidneys and have only specialized application, not appropriate here. Pleurisy root (*Asclepias tuberosa*) is perhaps the only exception. It dilates the renal arteries, but with very little possible toxicity.

- **Couchgrass** (*Triticum [Agropyron] repens*), tea.
- **Burdock** (*Arctium lappa* or *A. minus*), tea.
- **Shepherd's purse** (*Capsella pursa-pastoris*), tincture or tea (recently harvested herb only).
- **Chicory** (*Cichorum*), tea.
- **Mormon tea** (*Ephedra viridis, E. nevadensis,* etc.), tea (not to be confused with *Ephedra sinica* or other Asian species sold as Ma Huang).
- **Horsetail** (*Equisetum arvense* and others), tea.
- **Goldenrod** (*Solidago spp.*), tea.
- **Dandelion** (*Taraxacum spp.*), tea.
- **Nettles** (*Urtica dioica*), tea.
- **Cleavers** (*Galium aparine*), tea.
- **Asparagus root** (*Asparagus spp.*), tea or tincture.

- **Puncture vine** (*Tribulus terrestris*), tea or tincture.

5. ***Urinary Anti-inflammatories.*** These tend to diminish general inflammatory states such as occur with allergies. Although one usually associates allergies with sinus or intestinal problems, being in a state of hypersensitivity, with inflammatory or immunologic compounds carried in the blood itself, can manifest as urinary tract, bladder or urethral irritability. The herbs below show specific value when this happens.

- **Witch hazel** (*Hamamelis spp.*), tea or tincture.
- **Squaw vine** (*Mitchella repens*), tea.
- **Garden sage** (*Salvia officinalis*), tea or tincture.
- **Stone root** (*Collinsonia canadensis*), fresh root tincture.
- **Alfalfa** (*Medicago sativa*), tea or capsules.
- **Pygeum** (*Pygeum [Prunus] africana*), tea, tincture or capsules.
- **Butcher's broom** (*Ruscus aculeatus*) tea, tincture or capsules.
- **Saw palmetto** (*Serenoa spp.*), tincture or capsules.
- **Red clover** (*Trifolium pratense*), tea.
- **Chickweed** (*Stellaria media*), tea of recent plant or fresh plant juice.

6. ***Urinary Analgesics.*** These contain constituents that are excreted in the urine and thereby decrease pain. Although seemingly palliative, constant urination to relieve pain can diminish the tone of the bladder and cause excess stress on the urethra. Use of such an herbal analgesic can actually help heal a condition, while decreasing pain.

- **Yerba mansa** (*Anemopsis californica*), tea or tincture.
- **Marijuana** (*Cannabis sativa*), tea or tincture. (Yes, it is illegal to possess, but this may meet the standards for

legal medicinal use in California and Arizona. Besides, it's just an herb, with little toxicity, and it works.)

- **Meadowsweet** (*Filipendula spp.*), tea, tincture or capsule.
- **Kava kava** (*Piper methysticum*), tea, tincture or capsule.
- **Aspen** or **Poplar** (*Populus spp.*), tea, tincture or capsule. (White willow bark capsules can be used as a substitute.)

*7. Urinary Antispasmodics.* The urethra and bladder are both muscular organs, and, for many UTIs, there can be accompanying cramps, even involving the uterus, seminal vesicles and descending colon. In these cases, the following herbs may sometimes be necessary.

*General Use*

- **Catnip** (*Nepeta cataria*), tea or tincture.
- **Wood betony** or **Lousewort** (*Pedicularis spp.*), tea or tincture.
- **Skullcap** (*Scutellaria spp.*), tea or tincture (the more recently harvested the better).
- **Peony root** (*Paeonia spp.*), tincture (made with fresh herb is best).

*Industrial Strength*

- **Hydrangea** or **Seven Barks** (*Hydrangea arborescens*), tea or tincture.

You will find the specific references on each plant as well as dosages and preparation methods in the *Herbal Pharmacy* section, and some sample formulas in the *Herbal Formula* section. Still it's fun to put together your own formulas, and probably also more healing. If you can do your own growing and/or gathering of your herbs as well, that's best of all.

# *Interstitial Cystitis*

Interstitial cystitis is a chronic disorder of bladder function characterized by frequent and urgent urination and bladder and pelvic pain, aggravated as the bladder fills. Like fibromyalgia, chronic fatigue syndrome and multiple chemical sensitivities, it is yet another one of our chronic and subtle late-20th century health problems, whose causes include iatrogenesis, environmental factors, poor diet, and something akin to a cultural "spirit sickness." All of these disorders are prevalent in the industrialized world, with the U.S. topping the list with the most sufferers.

Even a decade ago, those with such disorders as Epstein-Barr and cytomegalovirus infections, as well as those with interstitial cystitis, were generally treated as if they were suffering from "yuppie burnout"—self-obsessed hypochondriacs who should simply get back to work and shut up. Since 90 percent of those with interstitial cystitis were and are women, the most frequent response was tranquilizers and other antianxiety agents. These women had "neurotic bladders," were probably neurotic themselves and were best dealt with by shunting them over to the garbage collectors in psychiatry. It took the work of a physician-sufferer, Vicky Ratner, stubbornly educating her profession and the public about the disorder, to finally start to get medical recognition of the disease. The organization she founded, the Interstitial Cystitis Foundation (ICF), estimates that, as of 1995, the average person sees *seven* physicians before the condition gets correctly diagnosed.

To quote the ICF:

> Interstitial Cystitis is generally caused by a chronic inflammation of the bladder wall and produces symptoms that wax and wane. Scientists aren't certain what triggers the inflammatory process; suspects include previous infections; unidentified substances in the urine; defects in the cells lining the bladder; disorders of nerve functions; activation of mast cells, which play an important role in allergic reactions; or a combination of these factors. Whatever the cause, the affected bladder wall is hypersensitive to stimulation, and the presence of even a small amount of urine causes it to contract. As a result, discomfort is almost constant during flares of interstitial cystitis; pain and pressure are relieved only temporarily after responding to each urge to urinate.

Although the condition can appear out of the blue in people who have had no urinary problems, it is more likely to occur in those who have endured several bouts with bladder disease. An estimated 70 percent of women with interstitial cystitis have a history of urinary tract infections and many report having had childhood bladder problems.

## TREATMENT PHILOSOPHY

Since interstitial cystitis is not a specific disease entity deriving from specific causes but an end result, like arthritis, that can be reached through many pathways, the best holistic approach is to first strengthen the metabolism through tonics and then start using specific therapeutics until something works . . . trial and error. It is very likely that an approach that helps now may gradually stop working in a few months, so having several approaches is preferable. Using herbs alone is less beneficial than combining botanicals with traditional Chinese Medicine (TCM), nutritional counseling and bodywork.

Medical procedures are similarly "pyramidal" . . . including water dilation of the bladder, instillation of DMSO, the use of tricyclic antidepressants, agents such as sodium pentosan polysulfate to alter the bladder mucosa; even, finally, various drastic resections, restructuring and even complete removal of the bladder.

## Single Herb Strategies

### Herbs That Improve the Quality of Bladder Mucosa

- **Marshmallow** or **Hollyhock** (*Althea officinalis* or *A. rosea*), 2 grams in tea, 4x a day as a suspended cold infusion. See p. 72.
- **Slippery elm bark** (*Ulmus rubra*), 2 grams in tea, 4x a day as a suspended cold infusion.
- **Yerba mansa root** (*Anemopsis californica*), 2 grams in tea, 4x a day as an infusion, hot or cold.

### Antispasmodic Herbs to Decrease Pain

- **Kava kava** (*Piper methysticum*), fresh root tincture, 30 to 50 drops in hot water, 4x a day.
- **Marijuana** (*Cannabis sativa*), tincture, 45 to 90 drops in hot water, 4x a day.

### Herbs to Use in Sitz Baths

- **Yerba mansa** leaf or root (*Anemopsis californica*), analgesic and antimicrobial.
- **Mormon tea** (*Ephedra viridis, E. nevadensis,* etc.), astringent (not to be confused with *Ephedra sinica* or other Asian species sold as Ma Huang).

- **Chickweed** (*Stellaria media*), cooling, mildly anti-inflammatory.
- **Anil del muerto** (*Verbesina encelioides*), strongly anti-inflammatory.

**Herbs to Use for Tissue Edema (in Sitz Baths)** These herbs contain coumarin, a vanilla-scented compound that is very useful in lessening the edema and puffiness caused by stretched capillary protein leakage.

- **Sweet clover** (*Melilotus spp.*).
- **Deer's tongue** (*Liatris odorata*).

**Other Helpful Herbs**

- **Psyllium seed** as a dietary supplement. It contains soluble fiber that helps sustain colon mucosa and usually lessens the general pelvic congestion that goes along with IC.
- **Echinacea angustifolia** or **E. pallida** to decrease tissue edema and damage.
- **Mullein root tea** (*Verbascum thapsus*) to strengthen trigone muscle in early stage incontinence.
- **Lobelia inflata,** fresh herb tincture as a parasympathomimetic antispasmodic, particularly useful for adrenalin stressed folks with IC.
- **Peony root** (*Paeonia albiflora* or *P. brownii*), fresh root tincture to decrease concurrent reproductive irritability and lessen the small muscular cramps that contribute to the pain of IC.

**Further Resources**

Interstitial Cystitis Association
P.O. Box 1553 Madison Square Station
New York, NY 10159-1553
212-979-6057 or 1-800-ICA-1626

# Kidney Stones

Kidney stones are one of the most common disorders of the urinary tract and one of the most painful disorders to afflict humans. It is estimated that ten percent of all people in the United States will have a kidney stone at some point in time, with men having three or four times as many as women.

Kidney stones are not a modern disease; archeologists have found evidence of kidney stones in an Egyptian mummy estimated to be more than 7,000 years old. Nonetheless, as with many other disorders that reflect contemporary stress and diet, the number of persons in the United States with kidney stones has been increasing over the past 30 years. Caucasians are more prone to kidney stones than are African-Americans, and although stones occur more frequently in men, the percentage of women who get kidney stones has also been increasing. Kidney stones strike most of these people between the ages of 20 and 40. Once a person gets more than one stone, he or she is more likely to develop others.

Most kidney stones pass out of the body without any intervention by a physician. Cases that cause lasting symptoms or other complications may be treated by various methods, and several newer procedures use sound waves and lasers, reducing the need for traditional invasive surgery to only a small percentage of cases.

## What Is a Kidney Stone?

A kidney stone develops from precipitated crystals that separate out from urine and build up on the inner surfaces of the kidney. Normally, urine contains substances that prevent or inhibit the crystals from forming. These are secreted by both the kidneys and the mucous membranes, in one of our body's many exquisitely balanced metabolic acts. These inhibitors do not seem to work for everyone. If the crystals remain small enough and do not clump or bind together, they will travel through the urinary tract and out of the body in urine without even being noticed.

Kidney stones can be formed from a variety of compounds; however, the most common type of stone contains calcium in combination with either oxalate or phosphate. These compounds are part of a person's normal diet and are important components in a variety of tissues, such as bones and muscles.

A less common type of stone is caused by infection in the urinary tract with bacteria that are capable of breaking down urea, a normal urine constituent. This type of stone is called a struvite or infection stone, and may sometimes form extensive "staghorn" concretions in the pelvis of one or both kidneys. Much less common are uric acid stones and the rare cystine stone.

Urolithiasis is the medical term used to describe stones occurring in the urinary tract. Other frequently used terms are urinary tract stone disease and nephrolithiasis. Doctors also use terms that describe the location of the stone in the urinary tract. For example, a ureteral stone (or ureterolithiasis) is a kidney stone found in the ureter. To keep things simple, I am using the term "kidney stones."

## What Causes Kidney Stones?

A stone can form only when urine is supersaturated with one or more of its constituent crystals, either from too much of that substance, or too little of the protective proteins from the urine and mucosa.

Supersaturation means that the concentration of a stone-forming salt, such as calcium oxalate, exceeds its solubility in urine. The substance "snows," much like when a 100-percent saturation of water in the air becomes rain or snow. The urine of most normal people is supersaturated with calcium oxalate, so, in principle, all people can form such stones. Normal urine is not supersaturated with uric acid, cystine or struvite.

Any conditions that raise calcium oxalate supersaturation raise the risk of calcium oxalate stones, and any conditions that lessen the urinary tract "emulsifiers" also raise the risk of these, and in fact, any stones.

Many disorders can raise the levels of both calcium and oxalates. Further, hyperparathyroidism, renal tubular acidosis, sarcoidosis, vitamin D intoxication and "idiopathic" hypercalciuria all are causes of hypercalciuria (elevated urine calcium). Elevated oxalates (or hyperoxaluria) may be due to overproduction from hereditary disorders of metabolism or be acquired from intestinal disease or diet.

The causes of diminished production of the protective urinary proteins is unknown, but in my opinion, the chronic skin and mucosal hyposecretion that results from adrenal stress as well as from certain decongestants and allergy medications can also contribute to kidney stones.

Doctors do not always know what causes a stone to form. While certain foods may promote stone formation in people who are susceptible, scientists do not believe that eating any specific food causes stones to form in people who are not susceptible.

A person with a family history of kidney stones may be more likely to develop stones. Urinary tract infections, kidney disorders such as cystic kidney diseases and metabolic disorders such as hyperparathyroidism are also linked to stone formation.

In addition, more than 70 percent of patients with the hereditary disease called renal tubular acidosis develop kidney stones.

Cystinuria and hyperoxaluria are two other rare inherited metabolic disorders that often cause kidney stones. In cystinuria, the kidneys produce too much of the amino acid cystine. Cystine does not dissolve in urine and can build up to form stones. With hyperoxaluria, the body produces too much of the salt oxalate. When there is more oxalate than can be dissolved in the urine, the crystals settle out and form stones.

Absorptive hypercalciuria occurs when the body absorbs too much calcium from food and empties the extra calcium into the urine. This high level of calcium in the urine causes crystals of calcium oxalate or calcium phosphate to form in the kidneys or urinary tract.

Other causes of kidney stones are hyperuricosuria (a disorder of uric acid metabolism), gout, excess intake of vitamin D, and urinary tract blockage. Some prescription diuretics and some calcium-based antacids may increase the risk of forming kidney stones by increasing calcium in the urine.

Calcium oxalate stones can also form in people with either ulcerative colitis or who have had intestinal bypass surgery. As mentioned above, struvite stones can form in people who have had a urinary tract infection.

## SYMPTOMS

Usually, the first symptom of a kidney stone is extreme pain. The pain often begins suddenly when a stone moves in the urinary tract, causing irritation or blockage. The usual symptoms are a sharp, cramping pain in the back and side in the area of the kidney or in the lower abdomen. Sometimes nausea and vomiting occur with this pain. Later, the pain may spread to the groin. Some people (such as myself) only feel deep restlessness with ill-defined abdominal aching.

Passing a kidney stone results in what is called referred pain. The pain is not the simple and well-defined distress of a broken finger or topical injury, with local nerve endings in the skin sending distress signals to the spinal cord and up to the brain. Referred pain derives from nerve impulses sent by the autonomic nervous system to the spinal cord nerves of the central nervous system. There are a variety of possible sensations that can occur, ranging from profound agony to an ill-defined distress somewhat similar to menstrual cramps or gas pain. Such referred pain is notoriously difficult to define at first. General abdominal pain in its early stages can derive from kidney stones, an ovarian cyst, appendicitis or under-cooked lentils . . . it all feels the same. Only as the inflammation progresses can one start to define where and what is causing the pain.

If the stone is too large to pass easily, the pain continues and becomes more of a lower back and flank phenomenon as the muscles in the wall of the ureters try to squeeze the stone along into the bladder. As a stone grows or moves, blood may be found in the urine. As the stone moves down the ureter closer to the bladder, a person may feel the need to urinate more often or feel a burning sensation during urination. A large stone may lodge briefly at the mouth of the urethra and finally induce sharp, local, "unreferred" pain.

For women, the passage out of the body is usually simpler; women tend to have a short and more resilient urethra. Having such a stone lodged midway in the penis of a male is a bit nightmarish.

If fever and chills accompany any of these symptoms,

an infection may be present. In this case, a doctor should be contacted immediately.

**Diagnosis**

The majority of stones, 70 to 80 percent, are composed mainly of calcium oxalate crystals; the rest are composed of calcium phosphate salts, uric acid, struvite (magnesium, ammonium and phosphate) or the amino acid cystine. Occasionally, stones injure kidneys and reduce their function by causing infection or obstruction, but most people with stones suffer only from the pain and rather self-limiting symptoms of the stone passage. In essence, kidney stones are a common cause of disease rather than of death or renal failure.

A diagnosis of kidney stones is not difficult in most people. The pain of stone passage, called renal colic, has easily recognized characteristics including location in the flank, sudden onset, extreme severity, radiation down the abdomen toward the groin, association with some blood in the urine and urinary symptoms of frequency, urgency and pain.

Relief immediately follows the stone passage . . . sometimes almost miraculously. Stone passage itself or radiographic evidence of the stone and its attendant urinary obstruction make the diagnosis certain.

## TREATING KIDNEY STONES WITH HERBS

Fortunately, the vast majority of kidney stones can be treated without surgery. Most kidney stones can pass through the urinary system with plenty of water and tea (2 to 3 quarts a day) to help move the stone along.

**Herbal Diuretics** that increase the volume of urine without increasing the wastes should be taken as tea. Those include:

- **Fenugreek** (*Trigonella foenum-graecum*).
- **Burdock** (*Arctium lappa* or *A. minus*).
- **Horsetail** (*Equisetum arvense* and others).
- **Couchgrass** (*Triticum [Agropyron] repens*).
- **Dandelion** (*Taraxacum spp.*).
- **Chicory root** (*Cichorum*).
- **Shepherd's purse** (fresh tincture, preferably).
- **Mormon tea** (*Ephedra viridis, E. nevadensis,* etc.).
- **Cleavers** (Galium aparine).
- **Nettles** (*Urtica dioica*).

Herbs that relax the smooth muscles of the ureters and/or bladder include:

- **Lobelia inflata** (fresh tincture, preferably).
- **Gravel root** (*Eupatorium purpureum*).
- **Hydrangea** or **Seven barks** (*Hydrangea arborescens*).
- **Wild yam** (*Dioscorea villosa*).

After the stone has passed, herbs that soothe the irritated mucosa as well as those that stop any bleeding should be taken. These include:

- **Marshmallow** or **Hollyhock** (*Althea officinalis* or *A. rosea*).
- **Corn silk** (*Zea mays*).
- **Yarrow** (*Achillea millefolium*).
- **Shepherd's purse** (fresh tincture, preferably).
- **Canadian fleabane** (*Conyza [Erigeron] canadense*).

*Note:* All of these herbs should be taken as a tea. See the *Materia Medica* section for specifics.

For hyperacidic anabolic individuals, and those with uric acid stones, the best herbs are generally burdock, dandelion and shepherd's purse, along with tonics for anabolic stress and changes in diet.

## PREVENTING KIDNEY STONES THROUGH LIFESTYLE CHANGES

A simple and most important lifestyle change to prevent stones is to drink more liquids. Water is best, although some of the safe diuretic teas listed above can be substituted periodically. A recurrent stone former should try to drink enough liquids throughout the day to produce at least two quarts of urine in every 24-hour period. This varies with body weight.

As a stone maker myself, this simple regimen of increasing fluid intake has stabilized my condition to a single stone every couple of years, passed with minimum discomfort using some fresh *Lobelia inflata* tincture. During the heat of the summer and when I sweat heavily, I increase my water intake accordingly. It makes a big difference.

Folks with too much calcium or oxalate in the urine may need to eat fewer foods containing calcium and oxalate. Although there is much emphasis given to calcium in our diet, those of us with a history of kidney stones generally need to back down a bit.

Not everyone will benefit from a low-calcium diet, however. Some who have high levels of oxalate in their urine may benefit from extra calcium in their diet. It may help to avoid food with added vitamin D and certain types of anticids that have a calcium base.

Those with kidney stones who take heavy regimens of nutritional supplements, with an emphasis on amino acids and glandulars, may find that these can contribute to the problem as well, since "one size fits all" is a philosophically bankrupt approach to health. Megavitamin approaches may be fine for those coming out of the long tunnel of chronic fatigue syndrome or multiple chemical sensitivities, but many nutritional approaches fail to allow for those of us who have imbalances in urine chemistry, renal function or lower urinary tract health. *Remember:* you have to pee out the metabolites of all these supplements. Sometimes moderation (and more water) is a better approach.

Those who have a very acid urine may need to eat less meat, fish and poultry. These foods increase the amount of acid in the urine.

**Prevention Guidelines**

- People who have a family history of stones are likely to develop stones themselves.
- People who have had more than one stone are likely to develop another.
- A good first step to prevent any type of stone is to drink plenty of liquids. Water is best.
- If a person is at risk for developing stones, a physician may perform certain blood and urine tests. These tests will determine which factors can be best altered to reduce the risk.
- Some patients will need medicines to prevent stones from forming. This is particularly important for staghorn or struvite stones.
- People with chronic urinary tract infections and stones will often need the stone removed if the doctor determines that the infection results from the stone's presence. Patients must receive careful follow-up to be sure that the infection has cleared.

**Foods and Drinks Containing Calcium and Oxalate**

Persons prone to forming calcium oxalate stones may need to cut back on certain foods on this list.

- apples
- asparagus
- beer
- beets
- berries
- black pepper
- broccoli
- cheese
- chocolate
- cocoa
- coffee
- cola drinks
- collards
- figs
- grapes
- ice cream
- milk
- oranges
- parsley
- peanut butter
- pineapples
- spinach
- Swiss chard
- rhubarb
- tea
- vitamin C
- yogurt

# The Herbal Pharmacy

Unless otherwise noted, the following herbs have no contraindications.

**Agrimony** *(Agrimonia spp.)*

*Part(s) used:* The aerial parts of the plant, gathered when in flower.

*Therapeutic effects:* Astringent, useful for the urinary tract and the intestinal tract.

*Preparations and dosages:* Standard infusion, 2 to 4 ounces as needed. Tincture [1:5, 50% alcohol, or fresh plant, 1:2], ¼ to 1 teaspoon as needed.

**Alfalfa** *(Medicago sativa)*

*Part(s) used:* The leaves, small stems and flowers.

*Therapeutic effects:* Mild and safe anti-inflammatory, alkalyzing tea for metabolic stress with acidic, concentrated urine, and a nutritionally significant tea for mineral deficiencies.

*Preparations and dosages:* Standard infusion as needed.

**Asparagus root** *(Asparagus spp.)*

*Parts(s) used:* The fresh or dried octopoidal rhizome.

*Therapeutic effects:* A simple volume diuretic, particularly useful with acidic, concentrated urine.

*Preparations and dosages:* Tincture [fresh, 1:2, dry, 1:5, 50% alcohol], 30 to 60 drops in water, 3x a day.

*Contraindications:* Not advisable for use by those with a history of nephritis. It can irritate weak kidneys.

**Aspen** or **Poplar** *(Populus spp.)*

*Part(s) used:* Bark of the tree or branches. Aspen outer bark is paper-thin and can be used along with the inner bark, but poplar has thick outer bark that must be removed.

*Therapeutic effects:* A source of salicylates, it is less irritating to the stomach than aspirin or willow bark as the absorption is slower and predominantly in the small intestine; this extended presence makes it useful for its effect on lower urinary tract inflammation.

*Preparations and dosages:* Strong decoction, 2 to 4 ounces, up to 4x a day when condition is acute. The tincture (1:5, 50% alcohol) can be used in 45 to 60 drop doses in a full cup of warm water.

*Contraindications:* Allergies to salicylates or aspirin analogues; use of anticoagulant drugs.

**Buchu** *(Agothasma* or *Barosma spp.)*

Part(s) used: Leaves.

*Therapeutic effects:* A traditional and effective aromatic urinary tract disinfectant.

*Preparations and dosages:* Cold infusion (rewarmed) 1 to 3 ounces. Tincture [1:5, 80% alcohol], 30 to 60 drops in water. Both forms to 4x a day.

*Contraindications:* Better for use in subacute/chronic UTI

as it may irritate acute stages. May color urine with plant pigments. Can aggravate nephritis.

**Burdock** *(Arctium lappa* or *A. minus)*

*Part(s) used:* The root (Fall of the first year or Spring of the second) and the seeds, winnowed from the chaffy seedheads.

*Therapeutic effects:* A volume diuretic and metabolic "cooler," particularly useful for anabolic stress and acidic, concentrated urine. It is a sodium leecher that also increases efficiency of uric acid excretion. Together with dandelion root, the perfect tonic for the overstressed individual.

*Preparations and dosages:* **Root**: Cold infusion, 2 to 4 ounces. Tincture [fresh root, 1:2, dry root, 1:5, 60% alcohol] 30 to 90 drops, all 3x a day. **Seed:** Tincture [1:5, 60% alcohol] 10 to 25 drops. Strong decoction, 1 to 2 ounces, both to 4x a day.

**Butcher's Broom** *(Ruscus aculeatus)*

*Part(s) used:* The root and rhizome.

*Therapeutic effects:* A tonic herb for capillary and lymphatic congestion, it is particularly helpful for bladder and urethral inflammation and aching.

*Preparations and dosages:* Dry tincture [1:5, 60% alcohol] 30 to 60 drops, 3x a day. Pharmaceutical preparations (European) are easier to get than the crude herb and more reliable for chronic vascular congestion.

**Canadian Fleabane** *(Conyza [Erigeron] canadense)*

*Part(s) used:* The whole flowering plant, stem and all.

*Therapeutic effects:* One of the best herbs for mucus membrane irritation, bleeding and discharges, pleasant tasting and devoid of toxicity. The tea is preferable.

*Preparations and dosages:* Standard infusion 2 to 4 ounces. Tincture (fresh plant, 1:2), 60 to 90 drops in a cup of warm water, all to 4x a day.

**Catnip** *(Nepeta cataria)*

*Part(s) used:* Flowering tops.

*Therapeutic effects:* An effective, if mild, antispasmodic for cramps of smooth muscle tubes, such as the intestinal tract, uterus and the lower urinary tract.

*Preparations and dosages:* Tincture [fresh herb 1:2, recent dry herb 1:5, 50% alcohol], ¼ to 1 teaspoon. Standard infusion, 2 to 6 ounces, all to 4x a day.

**Chickweed** *(Stellaria media)*

*Part(s) used:* Whole fresh plant.

*Therapeutic effects:* A soothing herb for pain with inflammation, either internally or topically; mildly diuretic.

*Preparations and dosages:* Fresh plant juice (1 to 2 tablespoons to 5x a day) or recently dried herb. Standard infusion, as needed. Tincture [fresh herb, 1:2, recent dry herb 1:5, 50% alcohol] as needed.

**Chicory Root** *(Cichorum)*

*Part(s) used:* Dried root.

*Therapeutic effects:* Related to both burdock and dandelion, it is a simple volume diuretic that also aids in excretion of retained sodium. It does, however, lack their subtler tonic effects on liver and kidney function.

*Preparations and dosages:* Strong decoction, 3 to 6 ounces, up to 4x a day.

**Cleavers** *(Galium aparine)*

*Part(s) used:* The fresh or dried herb in flower.

*Therapeutic effects:* A simple volume diuretic with mild astringent effects.

*Preparations and dosages:* Cold or standard infusion of dried herb, as needed. Fresh plant tincture [1:2] 1 to 2 teaspoons. Fresh plant juice, ½ to 1 teaspoon, all to 4x a day.

**Corn Silk** *(Zea mays)*

*Part(s) used:* The silk, either dried (straw-colored), dried and roasted (brownish purple) or fresh. Fans of corn silk seem to have strong opinions on this roasted-unroasted matter; I have found little difference myself.

*Therapeutic effects:* Soothing and analgesic to inflamed or injured urinary tract mucosa.

*Preparations and dosages:* Standard infusion, 4 to 6 ounces. Fresh silk tincture, [1:2], ½ to 1½ teaspoons in 8 ounces water, both to 3x a day.

**Couchgrass** *(Triticum [Agropyron] repens)*

*Part(s) used:* Roots and rhizomes.

*Therapeutic effects:* A volume diuretic. Although not as predictable a sodium leecher as either dandelion, burdock or chicory, it will sometimes work when they do not.

*Preparations and dosages:* Cold infusion, 2 to 4 fl. oz. Tincture [1:5, 50% alcohol] 30 to 60 drops. All forms to 5x a day.

**Cranesbill** or **Wild Geranium** *(Geranium spp.)*

*Part(s) used:* Root (traditional); whole plant (my preference).

*Therapeutic effects:* A simple and effective astringent and hemostatic, useful internally or topically.

*Preparations and dosages:* Tincture [1:5, 50% alcohol, 10% glycerin] in ½ to 1 teaspoon doses. Strong decoction, 1 to 4 ounces, both to 4x a day. The whole herb as a standard infusion as needed.

**Cubeb Berries** *(Piper cubeb)*

*Part(s) used:* Unripe dried berries.

*Therapeutic effects:* An aromatic disinfectant; like eucalyptus, it affects both the urinary tract and lungs.

*Preparations and dosages:* Tincture [1:5, 80% alcohol] 10 to 30 drops. Capsules, #00, 1 to 3. To 3x a day for up to a week.

*Contraindications:* Active inflammation, nephritis or a history of same. Cubeb berries scent the urine harmlessly. Extended use is discouraged and it may be contraindicated in a delicate pregnancy, just to be safe.

**Dandelion** *(Taraxacum spp.)*

*Part(s) used:* The root, gathered in the fall of the first year or the spring of the second year, preferably gathered from areas with distinct, cold winters. The leaf should be gathered in the spring, while still in active flowering. I prefer the root as a medicine.

*Therapeutic effects:* Like burdock, chicory and couchgrass, dandelion stimulates sodium excretion by the kidneys (with subsequent increased fluid excretion). This makes it very useful as a volume diuretic, particularly for sodium retention from kidney excess and anabolic stress. Like burdock it also helps cool an overheated metabolism. Because it stimulates bile secretions (without warming or irritating the liver), it is mildly laxative as well.

*Preparations and dosages:* Root: Tincture [fresh root, 1:2] ½ to 1 teaspoon. Strong decoction, 2 to 4 ounces, to 4x a day. Leaf as standard infusion, 3 to 6 ounces as needed.

**Deer's Tongue** *(Carphephorus [Liatris] odoratissimus)*

*Part(s) used:* Leaves.

*Therapeutic effects:* An herb to use topically or in a sitz bath when there is inflammatory congestion and edema.

*Preparations and dosages:* The tea as a sitz bath.

*Contraindications:* Recommended for external use only.

**Dong Quai** (cured *Angelica sinensis*)

*Part(s) used:* The cured root.

*Therapeutic effects:* Although it has no hormonal activity itself, dong quai stimulates the binding of existing steroid hormones, particularly estrogen and androgens.

*Preparations and dosages:* A single slice, 1/16 -1/8" thick a day, chewed and swallowed. Tincture [1:5, 70% alcohol] 5 to 20 drops to 3x a day. Capsules, #0, 1x to 3x a day.

*Contraindications:* Pregnancy, subclinical gonad or adrenalcortical hyperfunction, anabolic stress, hyptertension. Chewing the root or taking the tincture strongly stimulates gastric secretions and can cause indigestion in some folks.

**Echinacea Angustifolia** or **E. Pallida**

*Part(s) used:* The root (traditional), although I encourage the use of all parts of the plant, especially the flowers and stem. We squander incredible amounts of echinacea when we slavishly stick to roots only. I can make a liter of strong tincture using only five or six whole fresh plants.

*Therapeutic effects:* Echinacea helps to limit tissue damage and edema from trauma or extended inflammation. Although not an antibiotic, it does shorten the time the body takes to recognize foreign bodies and antigens and speeds up the formation of blood protein adherents that enable antibodies and T-cells to destroy these agents. In other words, it enhances body defenses.

*Preparations and dosages:* Tincture [fresh plant 1:2; dry plant, 1:5, 70% alcohol], 30 to 100 drops as needed. Cold infusion 2 to 6 ounces, all to 5x a day.

**Eucalyptus Leaves** *(Eucalyptus globulus)*

*Part(s) used:* Leaves.

*Therapeutic effects:* The oils from the tea are excreted in the urine and out the lungs as gases; in both regions the oils act to inhibit bacteria. The oils work topically as well.

*Preparations and dosages:* Standard infusion, 2 to 4 ounces, to 4x a day.

**Fenugreek** *(Trigonella foenum-graecum)*

*Part(s) used:* The seeds.

*Therapeutic effects:* A good volume diuretic with some anti-inflammatory and analgesic effects as well.

*Preparations and dosages:* Steep ½ ounce of seeds overnight in a pint of water. Then heat to nearly boiling, cool and strain. The syrupy tea that results should be drunk in 3 or 4 portions during the day. This may be continued for a week or more when backing down from high calcium-oxalate urine levels or a recent attack of kidney stones.

**Fireweed** or **Great Willow Herb** *(Epilobium angustifolium)*

*Part(s) used:* The aerial parts, gathered in early flower.

*Therapeutic effects:* An unsung but very effective antifungal, especially useful in dealing with candida flareups anywhere in the body. An herb that doesn't work so well in the petri dish but works well in people.

*Preparations and dosages:* The tea as needed.

**Garden Sage** *(Salvia officinalis)*

*Part(s) used:* The herb in flower.

*Therapeutic effects:* A good mucus membrane astringent, diminishing both inflammation and excess discharges; it is also mildly antimicrobial in the urine.

*Preparations and dosages:* Tincture [fresh, 1:2, dry, 1:5, 50% alcohol] 30 to 60 drops in hot water (diaphoretic) or cold water (tonic and diuretic). Cold infusion or strong decoction, 2 to 4 ounces, all as needed.

**Goldenrod** *(Solidago spp.)*

*Part(s) used:* The herb in early flower.

*Therapeutic effects:* A simple volume diuretic with some soothing effect.

*Preparations and dosages:* Standard infusion, 1 to 3 ounces every four hours.

**Gravel Root** *(Eupatorium purpureum)*

*Part(s) used:* The root and rhizome (although I have found that the whole plant is equally useful).

*Therapeutic effects:* An effective antispasmodic, analgesic and anti-inflammatory for the urinary tract, both for irritated bladder and urethra from a UTI and the pain of kidney stones (about to be or already passed). Extended hot baths while taking the herb helps greatly.

*Preparations and dosages:* Strong decoction, 2 to 4 ounces; tincture [fresh root or fresh plant, 1:2; dry root,

1:5, 60% alcohol] 30 to 90 drops in cup of warm water, all to 4x a day.

**Grindelia** *(Grindelia spp.)*

*Part(s) used:* The upper half of the flowering stems.

*Therapeutic effects:* Although a well-known expectorant herb, it is often overlooked as an excellent aromatic urinary tract disinfectant and analgesic.

*Preparations and dosages:* Tincture (fresh herb, [1:2]; dry herb, [1:5, 70% alcohol], 15–40 drops to 5x a day.

**Horsetail** *(Equisetum arvense and others)*

*Part(s) used:* The aerial parts.

*Therapeutic effects:* A simple diuretic that also helps strengthen inflamed, overworked or weak kidneys.

*Preparations and dosages:* Standard infusion, 2 to 4 ounces. Fresh plant tincture, 60 to 90 drops, both to 4x a day. As it is recommended for use in this book mostly as a diuretic, horsetail tea is better than the tincture (and less expensive).

*Contraindications:* None, although if gathered downstream from agribusiness, inorganic nitrates from fertilizers can cause horsetail to synthesize mildly toxic alkaloids which are not present under normal circumstances. Check with your herb source if unsure.

**Huckleberry** or **Blueberry** *(Vaccinium spp.)*

*Part(s) used:* The leaves with a few stems.

*Therapeutic effects:* A mild urinary tract antimicrobial devoid of tannins. It is also mildly soothing to urinary tract mucosa.

*Preparations and dosages:* Standard infusion of recent herb, 3 to 4 ounces, to 3x a day.

**Hydrangea** or **Seven Barks** *(Hydrangea arborescens)*

*Part(s) used:* Root (traditional); whole fresh plant (my preference).

*Therapeutic effects:* An effective antispasmodic, analgesic and anti-inflammatory for the urinary tract, both for irritated bladder and urethra from a UTI and especially the pain of passing kidney stones. Similar to gravel root, but it can be used as a tonic for long periods of time to strengthen the mucous membranes.

*Preparations and dosages:* Root: Cold infusion or strong decoction, 3 to 6 ounces, frequently. Tincture, [fresh plant, 1:2; dry root, [1:5, 50% alcohol], ½ to 1 teaspoon in water, up to 4x a day.

*Contraindications:* None that I have observed. Although some writers seem to think it can be toxic, in my experience it is not.

**Juniper Berries** *(Juniperus communis)*

*Part(s) used:* The berries (commercially available); the leaves (works fine but you need to gather them yourself).

*Therapeutic effects:* An aromatic disinfectant with mild but overrated diuretic effects. Milder agents usually work, but adding a bit of juniper to a formula where the UTI has been persistent and recurring will sometimes make it work.

*Preparations and dosages:* Berries: Tincture [1:5, 75% alcohol], 20 to 40 drops. Standard infusion of crushed berries, 2 to 3 ounces, to 3x a day. Leaves: Standard infusion, 2 to 4 ounces.

*Contraindications:* Renal disease, gastric inflammation,

pregnancy. For short-term use; may irritate the kidneys in time.

**Kava Kava** *(Piper methysticum)*

*Part(s) used:* The root and rhizome (although the whole herb has begun to enter the market).

*Therapeutic effects:* An excellent herb for urinary tract pain, particularly when it is sharp, burning, localized and induced by urinating, with the pain lingering a few minutes before subsiding. It is less useful for constant urethral pain.

*Preparations and dosages:* Tincture [fresh root 1:2; recent dry root 1:5, 60% alcohol] 30 to 90 drops. Cold infusion, 2 to 6 ounces, all to 4x a day.

*Contraindications:* None in these ranges of dosage, although with the advent in the health food market of concentrated high-potency pharmaceutical preparations from Europe, one could run the risk of stupefaction.

**Ladies Mantle** *(Alchemilla)*

*Part(s) used:* The dried herb.

*Therapeutic effects:* A simple, reliable urinary tract astringent.

*Preparations and dosages:* Standard infusion, as needed.

**Licorice Root** *Glycyrrhiza glabra* and others)

*Part(s) used:* Rhizomes, taproot.

*Therapeutic effects:* An herb primarily for kidney deficiency, with frequent urination, particularly in the evenings before bed, especially for those with constipation and allergies. It will also help lessen chronic urinary tract inflammation.

*Preparations and dosages:* Tincture [1:5, 50% alcohol] 3

to 60 drops. Strong decoction, 1 to 3 ounces, either to 3x a day.

*Contraindications:* It can cause sodium retention in certain people, including pregnant women.

**Lobelia** *(Lobelia Inflata)*

*Part(s) used:* The fresh plant.

*Therapeutic effects:* The premier antispasmodic, capable of lessening pain on urination and stopping the pain of stone passage in its tracks. The fresh plant tincture is an excellent nervine tonic for adrenalin stress or kidney deficiency.

*Preparations and dosages:* Fresh plant tincture [1:4] 5 to 20 drops up to 4x a day. Dry plant tincture (inferior) is best as an acetum tincture [dry herb 1:5 in vinegar] 10 to 20 drops, or used for local application. Seed: Tincture [1:5, 65% alcohol), 3 to 10 drops. Herb tea is especially nauseating, fresh herb or seed preparations only slightly.

*Contraindications:* Any disorders characterized by cholinergic or parasympathetic excess, such as an abnormally slow pulse, low blood pressure, etc. Despite a century and a half of conflict about the toxicity of lobelia (or lack thereof), frankly speaking, a few drops of the tincture could save your life. However, an ounce could end it. USE WITH CARE.

**Marijuana** *(Cannabis sativa)*

*Part(s) used:* Whole herb or flower "shake." Flowering tops are better, but surprisingly expensive.

*Therapeutic effects:* An antispasmodic and analgesic, particularly useful for sharp, almost unbearable pain on urination during the peak of a UTI episode.

*Preparations and dosages:* Tincture [fresh herb, 1:2; dry

herb, 1:5, 95% alcohol] 5 to 30 drops. Smokers need higher doses.

*Contraindications:* ILLEGAL TO POSSESS AT PRESENT (except for medical use only in California and Arizona, as of this writing).
For three decades I have failed to understand the point of the whole *Cannabis* brouhaha. Relatively devoid of toxicity, with a number of rather well-defined herbal uses, one day in the 1950s it was a prescription drug with a long history of use, the next day it was the bane of conservative America. In point of fact, marijuana is a useful herb with few physiologic side effects in *therapeutic* doses. Unfortunately, the main practical side effects are that you could get into a heap of trouble if you are caught with it.

**Marshmallow** or **Hollyhock**
*(Althea officinalis* or *A. Rosea)*

*Part(s) used:* The second- or third-year roots (marshmallow, the herb of commerce, is usually sold peeled). The leaves and flowers of both are also usable.

*Therapeutic effects:* This is probably the single most useful herb I know of for soothing the bladder, ureters and urethra membranes after recuperating from an infection, stone episode or a bout of interstitial cystitis. It also acts as an immunostimulant and often seems to improve the membrane health as well.

*Preparations and dosages:* Root: Cold infusion or fresh tincture [1:2] as needed. Herb: Cold infusion as needed.

**Meadowsweet** *(Filipendula spp.)*

*Part(s) used:* Herb in flower.

*Therapeutic effects:* This is a well-known European plant with distinct aspirin-like effects, and, like aspen, helps substantially as a urinary tract analgesic.

*Preparations and dosages:* Fresh tincture [1:2], 60 to 90 drops; dry-tincture [1:5, 50% alcohol], 90 to 120 drops; standard infusion, 3 to 6 ounces; all to 4x a day.

*Contraindications:* Should not be used by those who need to avoid aspirin-related compounds either because of medications they are taking (such as coagulation drugs) or because of salicylate reactions.

**Mormon Tea** *(Ephedra viridis, E. nevadensis,* etc.)

*Part(s) used:* The dried stems.

*Special considerations:* The following warning is usually not a problem, as mormon tea is carefully hand-harvested. However, DO NOT CONFUSE IT WITH CHINESE EPHEDRA (ma huang) which is native to the deserts of Asia and North Africa and contains various quantities of the alkaloids ephedrine and pseudoephedrine. Although useful after a fashion, Ma huang is a strong central nervous system stimulant. Mormon tea lack the alkaloids in Ma huang and, besides being a substantial source of calcium and silica, is primarily astringent and diuretic. The last thing you want is to drink a formula for cystitis that contains, instead of the native ephedra, the Chinese herb sold to you by mistake. That means you will still hurt, and be awake all night as well. Be aware: Many health food retailers don't know their bulk herbs as well as they should.

*Therapeutic effects:* A simple volume diuretic and astringent. Traditional usage considers Mormon tea strengthening to the kidneys and lower urinary tract; this does, in fact, seem to be the case. Like uva ursi, it makes a soothing and anti-inflammatory sitz bath. It is perhaps the greatest source of calcium of any safe herb tea.

*Preparations and dosages:* Standard infusion, as needed. Tincture is available, but it is preferable as tea when used as a volume diuretic.

**Mullein Root Tea** *(Verbascum thapsus)*

*Part(s) used:* The root, Fall of the first or Spring of the second year. The flowers and leaves have many other uses, but only the root is of importance for urinary tract uses.

*Therapeutic effects:* An effective tonic and strengthener for the urethra and the base of the bladder, useful in urethral swelling and congestion with incontinence.

*Preparations and dosages:* Root tincture (fresh, 1:2, dry 1:5, 50% alcohol), 45 to 60 drops. Strong decoction, 2 to 3 ounces, all forms to 4x a day.

**Myrrh Gum** or **Guggul** *(Commiphora spp.)*

*Part(s) used:* The dried resin.

*Therapeutic effects:* Myrrh is a strong disinfectant, astringent and immunostimulant, used topically or in small doses of the tincture for obstinate, chronic cystitis.

*Preparations and dosages:* Tincture [1:5, 95% alcohol], 5 to 20 drops. Capsules, #0, 1 to 2, both to 3x a day.

*Contraindications:* Myrrh is a strong stimulant to bone marrow synthesis of white blood cells, and thus may be contraindicated in liver disease, autoimmune or collagen diseases, pregnancy and lymphomas.

**Nettles** *(Urtica dioica)*

*Part(s) used:* The leaf, preferably picked in late spring and early summer, before complete flowering.

*Therapeutic effects:* A fine volume diuretic with some anti-inflammatory and astringent effects. Nettles tea is one of the best teas to supply electrolytes and increase blood buffers for waste transport.

*Preparations and dosages:* Cold or standard infusion, as needed.

**Oregon Grape** *(Mahonia [Berberis] spp.)*

*Part(s) used:* The root (traditional) although the stems and foliage can be substituted with little loss in value.

*Therapeutic effects:* A stimulant to liver function and protein metabolism, Oregon grape is especially helpful to take along with dietary changes to increase protein and lipid consumption. This is often necessary for those with adrenalin stress, a chronic high glycemic index diet and overt kidney deficiency.

*Preparations and dosages:* Tincture [fresh root or whole plant, 1:2; dry root, 1:5, 50% alcohol] 10 to 60 drops. Cold infusion, 1 to 3 ounces. Capsules, #00, 1 to 3. All to 3x a day.

*Contraindications:* Acute inflammation, pregnancy, liver disease and hyperthyroid conditions.

**Pau D'Arco** *(Tabebuia spp.)*

*Part(s) used:* The bark.

*Therapeutic effects:* A very effective antifungal for those with chronic candida. One of the best antioxidant herbs.

*Preparations and dosages:* Cold infusion, 2 to 4 ounces to 3x a day. Tincture [1:5, 50% alcohol], ½ to 1 teaspoon to 4x a day.

**Peony Root** *(Paeonia spp.)*

*Part(s) used:* Fresh, dried or slightly cured tubers (Chinese peony).

*Therapeutic effects:* One of the better herbal antispasmodics, particularly useful for recurring cramps of small smooth muscles and sphincters as differentiated from the usual wavelike cramps associated with the colon, uterus or ureters.

*Preparations and dosages:* Tincture [fresh root 1:2; dry root, 1:5, 60% alcohol], 10 to 25 drops up to 4x a day. Cold infusion, 1 to 2 ounces. Capsules, #00, 2 to 3 at a time.

*Contraindications:* None that I know of, although it is a potent enough therapeutic that there could be synergies with prescription opiates and analgesics.

**Pipsissewa** *(Chimaphila umbellata)*

*Part(s) used:* The aerial parts.

*Therapeutic effects:* A relative of uva ursi, pipsissewa has the same antimicrobial action, but without the high tannin content. Therefore it can be used for longer periods of time. Uva ursi and manzanita, the more abundant plants, should be used for the usual short-lived UTI; pipissewa for obstinant or long-term tonic use.

*Preparations and dosages:* Tincture [fresh plant, 1:2; dry plant, 1:5, 50% alcohol), 20 to 50 drops. Standard infusion 4 to 8 ounces, both to 4x a day.

**Pleurisy Root** *(Asclepias tuberosa)*

*Part(s) used:* The fresh or dried root.

*Therapeutic effects:* Pleurisy root mildly dilates the blood vessels to the nephrons, thereby increasing the volume of urine produced. It is a volume diuretic particularly useful for the person with kidney excess. Otherwise, it stimulates secretions in general and may help the kidney-deficient person with frequent urination, constipation, seemingly weak lungs and dry skin by shifting fluids to the skin, lungs and intestinal tract.

*Preparations and dosages:* Cold infusion, 2 to 4 ounces. Tincture [fresh, 1:2; dry, 1:5, 50% alcohol] 30 to 90 drops. Capsules, #00, 1 to 3, all to 3x a day.

*Contraindications:* Pregnancy, with heart medications and wherever a parasympathomimetic or vagus nerve stimulant is inappropriate, such as abnormally slow pulse and anticholinergic drug use.

**Pygeum** *(Pygeum [Prunus] africanum)*

*Part(s) used:* The bark.

*Therapeutic effects:* Although widely used in Europe for prostate difficulties, usually combined with saw palmetto, pygeum is, by itself, an efficient urinary tract soother and anti-inflammatory.

*Preparations and dosages:* 2 to 6 grams a day, taken in capsules or mixed with enough honey to make into "pills" and eaten. The whole bark is hard to find in commerce, but the European pharmaceutical preparations are easy to find in American health food stores and many pharmacies.

**Red Clover** *(Trifolium pratense)*

*Part(s) used:* The flowering upper branches, leaf, stem and blossoms picked before browning and dried quickly.

*Therapeutic effects:* A mineral-heavy tea with good, mild, long-term anti-inflammatory effects on the kidneys and lower urinary tract and for chronic inflammation in general.

*Preparations and dosages:* Standard infusion or strong decoction, 4 to 6 ounces to 3x a day. Some herbalists feel that bringing red clover to a very brief boil makes for better solubility, even though leaf and flower herb teas are normally only steeped.

**Rose Buds** *(Rosa spp.)*

*Part(s) used:* The buds or petals.

*Therapeutic effects:* A pleasant astringent tea for the urinary tract and upper intestinal tract.

*Preparations and dosages:* Standard infusion, 2 to 4 ounces, as needed.

**Rosemary** *(Rosmarinus spp.)*

*Part(s) used:* Leaves.

*Therapeutic effects:* Like sage, a mild astringent and antimicrobial for the urinary tract.

*Preparations and dosages:* Standard infusion 2 to 4 ounces, to 4x a day.

*Contraindications:* None, although the strong taste can cause mild indigestion.

**Saw Palmetto** *(Serenoa spp.)*

*Part(s) used:* The mature fruit.

*Therapeutic effects:* Although a well-known herb for prostate problems, it is also a very useful herb for diminishing pain and urethral irritation when urinating.

*Preparations and dosages:* Tincture [fresh berry, 1:2; dry berry, 1:5, 80% alcohol] 30 to 90 drops. Standard infusion, 2 to 4 ounces. All forms to 3x a day. I would avoid the many forms of saw palmetto sold by various brand names and in various formulas. Most derive from European pharmaceutical extracts, and cost far more than good herb or tincture in commerce.

**Shepherd's Purse** *(Capsella bursa-pastoris)*

*Part(s) used:* Whole plant.

*Therapeutic effects:* One of the queens of urinary tract herbs, Shepherd's Purse is a volume diuretic, astringent and soothing herb for irritated mucosa and is helpful in stimulating uric acid excretion from the kidneys. It is particularly important as a preventive for those who form urate stones.

*Preparations and dosages:* Tincture (fresh plant, 1:2; recent dry plant, 1:5, 50% alcohol] 20 to 60 drops. Standard infusion of recent plant, 2 to 4 ounces. All forms to 5x a day.

*Contraindications:* Although theoretically a cholinergic and bradycardic plant, it really seems quite harmless in actual usage. Best to avoid in pregnancy, since shepherd's purse has the distinct potential to heighten oxytocin binding. It is, therefore, a widely used birthing herb.

**Skullcap** *(Scutellaria spp.)*

*Part(s) used:* Flowering herb.

*Therapeutic effects:* An effective analgesic for pain caused by nerve irritability.

*Preparations and dosages:* Herb: Tincture [fresh plant, 1:2, recent dry plant, 1:5, 50% alcohol] 20 to 60 drops. Standard infusion of recent herb, 2 to 6 ounces. All to 3x a day. Bad taste alert!

*Contraindications:* Probably should not be combined with other drug depressants or where a stronger approach is needed. Since you would presumably use a fresh preparation, you may experience a harmless temporary anesthetizing of the lips, fingers or toes. The herb's bitterness can induce gastric irritation in a few folks as well. Probably perfectly safe in pregnancy.

**Slippery Elm bark** *(Ulmus rubra)*

*Part(s) used:* Inner bark.

*Therapeutic effects:* A soothing demulcent for inflamed membranes, used either internally or topically.

*Preparations and dosages:* 2 grams in tea, 4x a day as a suspended cold infusion.

**Squaw Vine** *(Mitchella repens)*

Part(s) used: Whole herb (fresh is best).

*Therapeutic effects:* Astringent and tonic to the surface membranes of the reproductive organs and the lower urinary tract.

*Preparations and dosages:* Herb: Tincture [fresh plant, 1:2; dry plant, 1:5, 50% alcohol], ½ to 1 teaspoon to 3x a day. Standard infusion, 2 to 4 ounces to 4x a day.

**Stone Root** *(Collinsonia canadensis)*

*Part(s) used:* Fresh root or fresh whole plant (the dried root is traditional, but quite inferior).

*Therapeutic effects:* A particularly good tonic and astringent for chronically inflamed membranes, particularly when they alternate from time to time between sharp pain (red and hot) and dull, aching (congested and cold).

*Preparations and dosages:* Tincture [fresh plant or fresh root, 1:2], 15 to 30 drops to 3x a day.

*Contraindications:* Episodic hypertension, struvite kidney stones. Excess use can cause loose stools.

**Sweet Clover** *(Melilotus spp.)*

*Part(s) used:* The whole herb, preferably gathered in late spring.

*Therapeutic effects:* Mainly used for its coumarin content and pleasant vanilla-like scent, here sweet clover is recommended as a sitz bath for engorged and edemic tissues, particularly in interstitial cystitis.

*Preparations and dosages:* Standard infusion, at least 8 ounces in a sitz bath, as needed.

**Uva Ursi** or **Manzanita** *(Arctostaphylos spp.)*

*Part(s) used:* The dried leaves.

*Therapeutic effects:* A strong and reliable urinary tract antimicrobial. Not irritating to the kidneys as some aromatics are, its use is still limited to several days at a time because of its high tannin content.

*Preparations and dosages:* Standard infusion, 3 to 4 ounces to 3x a day. Tincture [1:5, 50% alcohol], 30 to 60 drops in 8 ounces of water, to 3x a day. For sitz bath, 8 to 12 ounces standard infusion added to warm bath water; sit in it morning and evening.

*Contraindications:* I usually recommend its use for no more than 3 to 4 days. Avoid during pregnancy. Uva Ursi's astringency has been implicated in vasoconstriction of the blood vessels of the uterus that nurture the placenta.

**Wild Yam** *(Dioscorea villosa)*

*Part(s) used:* Dried roots and rhizomes are found in general commerce, but, as is so often the case, the tincture of the fresh roots is far stronger.

*Therapeutic effects:* An effective traditional antispasmodic for rhythmic cramps of smooth muscle tubes such as the intestinal tract, bile ducts, uterus and ureters.

*Preparations and dosages:* Tincture [fresh root, 1:2; dry root, 1:5, 60% alcohol], 30 to 100 drops, to 4x a day. Cold infusion, 2 to 4 ounces to 4x a day.

Note: This is not Mexican yam (or Mexican wild yam); it contains no hormonal "precursors," no estrogen and no progesterone; nor does Mexican yam, for that matter. However, many "wild yam" products on the market do contain pharmaceutically manufactured "Natural Progesterone, U.S.P.," and others combine wild yam with other herbs and nutrients. Wild yam is a preeminent smooth muscle relaxant and antispasmodic herb. And that's all it is.

**Witch Hazel** *(Hamamelis spp.)*

*Part(s) used:* Leafing branches (less harmful to the plant), root and stem bark.

*Therapeutic effects:* A good astringent and soothing herb with distinct tonic effects on congested venous circulation, the type of aching pain that follows acute heat with sharp pain.

*Preparations and dosages:* Tincture [fresh herb, 1:2], 30 to 60 drops to 4x a day. Bark: Serviceable as standard decoction, 2 to 3 ounces to 4x a day.

**Wood Betony** or **Lousewort** *(Pedicularis spp.)*

*Part(s) used:* The herb in flower.

*Therapeutic effects:* A useful muscle relaxant for overexertion, excitation and the physical irritability from early stages of illness or extended pain.

*Preparations and dosages:* Standard infusion, 4 to 8 ounces. Tincture [fresh plant, 1:2; dry plant, 1:5, 50% alcohol] 60 to 90 drops. All to 3x a day.

*Contraindications:* A splendid muscle relaxant, all that one need worry about is that the herb not be gathered from host plants that have their own toxic constituents, such as mountain senecio or one of the mildly toxic legumes, such as mountain pea (*Thermopsis*). The wood betonies take up these constituents (when parasitic), and you have a remedy that is both itself and its host.

**Yarrow** *(Achillea millefolium)*

*Part(s) used:* Flowering plant.

*Therapeutic effects:* A good tea or tincture for inflamed membranes with mucus discharge or bleeding.

*Preparations and dosages:* Tincture [fresh 1:2, dry 1:5, 50% alcohol] 10 to 40 drops. Standard infusion, 2 to 4 ounces.

**Yerba Mansa** *(Anemopsis californica)*

*Part(s) used:* The root is most widely used and generally is all that is used in commerce. Although the leaves are serviceable, they lose potency rather more quickly than the root and are only practical if you are in a position to gather the plant yourself and use them right away.

*Therapeutic effects:* A remarkable little swamp plant for the Southwest, it is antimicrobial, astringent, soothing and anti-inflammatory and helps to remove acid wastes through the kidneys.

*Preparations and dosages:* Tincture [fresh root, 1:2; dry root, 1:5, 60% alcohol] 20 to 60 drops to 5x a day. Cold infusion, 2 to 4 ounces similarly. Herb: Standard or cold infusion as needed.

*Contraindications:* None known, although it can cause slight drowsiness in a few people.

**Yerba Santa** *(Eriodictyon californica* or *angustifolia)*

*Part(s) used:* Flowering tops.

*Therapeutic effects:* Like grindelia, yerba santa is best known as a lung and bronchial herb, but it is an effective and safe aromatic disinfectant for the urinary tract and is particularly useful for recurring, obstinate UTIs.

*Preparations and dosages:* Tincture [fresh herb, 1:2, dry herb, 1:5, 75% alcohol] 20 to 30 drops, to 5x a day. Standard infusion, 2 to 4 ounces as needed.

# *Preparation Methods*

## Teas

- 1 ounce of herb in a quart (32 fluid ounces) of water or
- ½ ounce of herb in a pint (16 fluid ounces) of water or
- ¼ ounce of herb in a cup (8 fluid ounces) of water

### Cold Infusion

After premoistening the herb, wrap 1 ounce (dry weight) in cloth and suspend it in 1 quart of water (by volume) at room temperature, overnight. Squeeze out the herb into the tea in the morning and add enough water to bring it back to 1 quart.

### Standard Infusion

Boil 1 quart water, remove from heat, and steep 1 ounce (by weight) of the herb in the water for 20 to 30 minutes. Strain and pour sufficient water through the herb in the strainer to return the volume of tea to 1 quart.

### Strong Decoction

Combine 1 quart water with 1 ounce of herb (by weight), bring slowly to a boil, continue for ten minutes, cool until warm and strain. Pour additional water through the herb to return the volume to 1 quart.

A weak decoction is made the same way, but use half

as much herb (½ ounce) in the same volume of water (1 quart).

Comments. Except for the weak decoction, the above teas end up with an ounce (2 tablespoons) having the constituents of a gram of herb. If my dosage recommends 4 ounces of strong decoction and you only want a single dose, use 4 grams of herb or divide an ounce of herb into eight equal parts and use one part for the tea. Do not make more than a day's worth of tea at one time.

## Sitz Baths

The simplest way is to add ½ to 1 ounce of the herb to 2 quarts of water, bring to a boil, remove from the heat and allow to steep and cool for 30 minutes. Add this to a half-bath of fairly warm water (deep enough to cover the hips). You will need to stay in the bath at least 30 minutes, adding some hot water as necessary. If it is cold outside, heat up the bathroom first; it doesn't help to get warm below if you are getting cold above.

There are plastic and metal tubs specifically designed for sitz baths, but it can be a delicate balance between getting the right temperature after adding the tea water, and not splashing the water all over after you sit in it. You can halve the amount of herb used for one of these little tubs, but I would suggest putting the tub in the bathtub before sitting in it to catch the overflow. Personally, I like the first method.

## Tinctures

### Fresh Plant Tincture

One part by weight of the fresh chopped herb is steeped

for 7 to 10 days in two parts by volume of grain alcohol (190 proof or 95% ethanol), and pressed or squeezed out. There is no reason to blend or shake this maceration; the tincture is formed passively as a result of dehydration. Ethanol draws out all plant constituents that contain water, leaving only cellulose and dead tissue behind.

**Dry Plant Tincture**

If the Herbal Pharmacy section calls for a [1:5, 60% alcohol] tincture, it means this: your solvent is 60% alcohol and 40% water (the water is presumed), and one part of herb by weight has been steeped in five parts by volume of solvent.

Example: Take 4 ounces of dried "cut and sifted" kava kava root, and grind and sift it down to a fairly consistent coarse powder. The 4 ounces (1 part) is then mixed with 20 ounces of solvent (5 parts). The solvent is 60% alcohol, the rest water, so you mix 12 ounces of ethanol and 8 ounces of water to get the final volume. Mix both together in a closed jar and shake the mixture up for a couple of minutes twice a day.

After 10 to 14 days of this, let the mixture set unshaken another day, pour off the clear tincture from the top and squeeze as much out of the sediment as your press or wrists allow.

**A cautionary note:** A few years ago the FDA decided that the term "tincture" implied drug intent and has, from time to time, forbade its use in labeling herbal extracts. That means that many manufacturers make tinctures but may not call them tinctures. Instead, you are faced with such terms as "extract," "tea extract" and even "herb drops."

The better herb manufacturers list the strength of the preparation, and you will find such definitions as "1:5" or "20%" on the label. Without any but voluntary standardization, some herb manufacturers follow the tried and true marketing ploy of making unique extracts that are "standardized," "chelated," "double-extracted" and so on. Tinctures were official methods of herb manufacturing, and the strengths I have recommended reflect former pharmaceutical standards and the majority of current manufacturing strengths. Many good sources exist, and some of the proprietary, nonstandard extracts are also well made.

Proper labeling should include the percentage of alcohol (at least 45% is needed to tincture properly), the strength of the extract (either listed as 1:5 or 1:2 or 20%, etc.), what part of the plant was used, and whether the herb was tinctured while fresh or dried. This is the moral minimum, and good herb tincture or extract makers label their products in this fashion.

You are usually better off using tinctures that reflect generic preparation methods and that are labeled accordingly.

# *Herbal Formulas*

**Kidney Deficiency Tincture Formula**

| | |
|---|---|
| Licorice root | 2 parts |
| Shepherd's purse | 2 parts |
| Siberian ginseng | 2 parts |
| Dong quai | 1 part |

Combine. Take 60 drops (2 squirts) 3x a day in a bit of warm water.

**Kidney Excess Tea Formula**

| | |
|---|---|
| Burdock root | 2 parts |
| Dandelion root | 2 parts |
| Pleurisy root | 1 part |
| Siberian ginseng | 1 part |

Combine the four herbs (based on weight), boil ½ ounce of the formula in a pint of water (a strong decoction), and drink ⅓ of the strained tea in 3 portions during the day.

**All Purpose Urinary Tincture**

| | |
|---|---|
| Buchu leaves | 3 parts |
| Juniper Berries | 2 parts |
| Yerba Mansa | 2 parts |
| Pipsissewa | 2 parts |
| Saw palmetto | 1 part |

Mix as tinctures or make 1:5, with 65% alcohol. Use 30 to 60 drops (1 or 2 squirts) in 8 ounces of water 3 to 4 times a day. A general diuretic and antimicrobial for water retention and mild urinary tract infections.

**Alkalinizing Tea**

| | |
|---|---|
| Nettle leaf | 1 part |
| Red clover tops | 1 part |
| Alfalfa | 1 part |
| Horsetail (optional) | (1 part) |

Drink the hot or cold tea freely. If under metabolic stress, you might even use the tea as your main liquid. Good for acid urine, uric acid kidney stones, post-op recovery, PMS acidity and as part of an interstitial cystitis regimen.

# *Herb Sources*

There are many more sources than I've listed here, but these are some that I have worked with and will vouch for.

Blessed Herbs
109 Barre Plains Road, Oakham, MA 01068.
800-489-4372, 508-882-3839, FAX: 508-882-3755.

Eclectic Institute Inc.
14385 SE Lusted Rd., Sandy, OR 97055.
503-668-4120, 800-332-4372, FAX: 503-668-3227.
Retail Information: 888–799–4372

eclectic-institute@worldnet.att.com
http://www.eclecticherb.com/

Frontier Herbs
Box 299, Norway, IA 52318.
800-669-3275.
http://www.frontierherb.com/

The Herb Pharm
Williams, OR 97544.
541-846-6262, 800-599-2392.
HerbPharm@aol.com

The Herbalist
2106 N.E. 65th, Seattle, WA 98115.
206-523-2600, 800-694-3727.
theherbalist@theherbalist.com
http://theherbalist.com/

Herbalist and Alchemist
P.O. Box 553, Broadway, NJ 08808.
908-689-9020.

Herbs Etc.
1345 Cerrillos Rd, Santa Fe, NM 87505.
888-694-3727.
herbsetcmo@aol.com

Turtle Island Herbs
2825 Wilderness Place, Boulder, CO 80301.
303-442-2215, 800-684-4060.
island@earthenet.net

Vitality Works
126 Quincy N.E., Albuquerque, NM 87108.
505-268-9950.
vitality@rt66.com

Winter Sun Trading Co.
107 N. San Francisco, Flagstaff, AZ 86001.
602-774-2884.
wintersn@primenet.com
http://www.wintersun.com

# *Recommended Reading*

Several of these are available on the internet and are so listed.

*BOTANY*

Benson, Lyman, and Robert A. Darrow, *Trees and Shrubs of the Southwestern Deserts,* 3d ed. Tucson, Ariz.: University of Arizona Press, 1981.

Elias, Thomas S., *The Complete Trees of North America.* New York: Van Nostrand Rheinhold, 1980.

Hickman, James C., Ed., *The Jepson Manual: Higher Plants of California.* Berkeley, Calif.: University of California Press, 1993.

Ivey, Robert DeWitt, *Flowering Plants of New Mexico, 2d ed.* Albuquerque, N.M.: Robert DeWitt Ivey, 1986.

Jepson, Willis *Manual of the Flowering Plants of California.* Berkeley, Calif.: University of California Press, 1960.

Kearney, Thomas, and Robert Peebles, *Arizona Flora.* Berkeley, Calif.: University of California Press, 1964.

Nelson, Ruth Ashton, Revised by Roger L. Williams, *Handbook of Rocky Mountain Plants, 4th ed.* Niwot, Colo.: Roberts Rinehart Publishers, 1992.

Ricket, Harold W., *Wild Flowers of the United States.* New York: McGraw-Hill Book Company, 1973.

Spellenberg, Richard, *The Audubon Society Field Guide to North American Wildflowers* (Western). New York: Alfred A. Knopf, 1979.

Vines, Robert A., *Trees, Shrubs and Woody Vines of the Southwest.* Austin, Tex.: University of Texas Press, 1960.

Willis, J. C., *A Dictionary of the Flowering Plants and Ferns.* Cambridge, England: Cambridge University Press, 1988.

### *ALTERNATIVE MEDICINE AND HERBALISM*

Culbreth, David, *A Manual of Materia Medica and Pharmacology, 1927.* Reprint. Portland, Oregon: Eclectic Medical Publications, 1983. Available at http://chili.rt66.com/hrbmoore/HOMEPAGE/HomePage.html.

Duke, James, *Handbook of Medicinal Herbs.* Boca Raton, Fla.: CRC Press, 1986.

*Phytochemical Constituents of GRAS Herbs and Other Economic Plants.* Boca Raton, Fla.: CRC Press, 1992.

Ellingwood, Finley, *American Materia Medica, 1917.* Reprint. Portland, Ore.: Eclectic Medical Publications, 1983.

Felter, H. Wicks, *Eclectic Materia Medica, 1919.* Reprint. Portland, Oregon: Eclectic Medial Publications, 1983. Available at http://chili.rt66.com/hrbmoore/HOMEPAGE/HomePage.html., and John U. Lloyd, *Kings American Dispensatory, 2 vols.* Portland, Oregon: Eclectic Medical Publications, 1983.

Foster, Steven, and James A. Duke, *A Field Guide to Medicinal Plants.* Boston: Houghton Mifflin, 1990.

Grieve, Maud, *A Modern Herbal. 2 vols. 1931.* Reprint. New York: Dover Publications, 1971. Available at http://www.bontanical.com/botanical/mgmh/mgmh.html

Harper-Shrove, F., *Prescriber and Clinical Repertory of Medicinal Herbs.* Devon, England: Health Science Press, 1952.

Hocking, George M., *A Dictionary of Terms in Pharmacognosy.* Springfield, Ill.: Thomas, 1955.

Kay, Margarita Artschwager, *Healing with Plants in the American and Mexican West.* Tucson, Ariz.: University of Arizona Press, 1996.

Lewis, Walter H., and Memory P. F. Elvin-Lewis, *Medical Botany.* New York: John Wiley, 1977.

Lloyd, John Uri, *Elixirs and Flavoring Extracts.* New York: William Wood, 1892. Available at http://chili.rt66.com/hrbmoore/HOMEPAGE/HomePage.html

Martinez, Maximo, *Las Plantas Medicinales de Mexico, 4th ed.* Mexico City: Botas, 1959.

Millspaugh, Charles, *American Medicinal Plants, 1892.* Reprint. New York: Dover Publications, 1974.

Moore, Michael, *Medicinal Plants of the Mountain West.* Santa Fe, N.M.: Museum of New Mexico Press, 1979.

———. *Medicinal Plants of the Desert and Canyon West.* Santa Fe, N.M.: Museum of New Mexico Press, 1989.

———. *Los Remedios: Traditional Herbal Remedies of the Southwest.* Santa Fe, New Mexico: Red Crane Books, 1990.

———. *Medicinal Plants of the Pacific West.* Santa Fe, N.M.: Red Crane Books, 1993.

Pizzorno, Joseph E. Jr. & Murray, Michael T. *A Textbook of Natural Medicine.* John Bastyr College Publications, Seattle, WA, 1985-present (updated quarterly). Parts are available at http://www.healthy.net/library/books/textbook/index.html

Uphof, J. C., *Dictionary of Economic Plants, 2d ed.* Lehre, Germany: J. Cramer, 1968.

## INTERNET RESOURCES

Rather than a long list of single resources, these are several primary link resources for the WWW (World Wide Web), together with several specific web sites that provide botanical, medical or herbal information.

The Internet Directory for Botany
http://www.helsinki.fi/kmus/botmenu.html

Botany: Guide to Internet Resources
http:/www.ualberta.ca/~slis/guides/botany/botany1.htm
Soaring Bear's Science Homepage
http://ellington.pharm.arizona.edu/~bear/index.html
Phytochemical and Ethnobotanical Databases
http://www.ars-grin.gov/~ngrlsb/
National Plants Database Access Page
http://trident.ftc.nrcs.usda.gov/plants/plntmenu.html
Biota of North America Program
http://trident.ftc.nrcs.usda.gov/plants/staselec.html
The Ethnobotany Cafe on the Web
http://countrylife.net/ethnobotany/
AANP: American Association of Naturopathic Physicians
http://www.pandamedicine.com

*And some sites dealing with herbal medicine:*
Michael Moore-SW School of Botanical Medicine
http://chili.rt66.com/hrbmoore/HOMEPAGE/Home Page.html
I have photographs of the plants used in this book (and 1,400 more)
The American Herbalists Guild.
http://www.healthy.net/herbalists/Index.html
Henriette's Herbal Homepage
http://sunsite.unc.edu/herbmed/
Herb Research Foundation:
http://www.herbs.org
HerbalGram Magazine
http://www2.outer.net/herbalgram/abc_herbalgram.html
Herbal Hall
http://www.herb.com/herbal.htm
herbnet
http://www.herbnet.com/
PhytoNet
http://www.exeter.ac.uk/phytonet
Robyn's Recommended Reading
http://www.herb.com/robyn.htm

# *APPENDIX: Glycemic Index*

The lower the number, the more slowly the food is utilized as blood sugar (and the longer it lasts); the higher the number, the more rapidly absorbed (and the more it jangles metabolism and the kidneys).

Most meats and fish are low in carbohydrates, and generally have little bearing on the basic purpose of the glycemic index which is to make sure there is a sound balance between the release of sugar into the bloodstream from diet and the release of fuel and sugar into the bloodstream from the liver. This in turn prevents excessive reliance on insulin and adrenalin for emergency blood sugar control.

| **RATING** | **FOOD ITEM** |
|---|---|
| **110** | **Maltose** |
| **100** | **Glucose** |
| **98** | **White potato, baked** |
| **97** | **Parsnips** |
| **92** | **Carrots** |
| **87** | **Honey** |
| **80** | **Potato, instant mashed** |
| **80** | **Cornflakes** |
| **72** | **Whole wheat bread** |
| **72** | **White rice** |
| **69** | **White bread** |
| **68** | **Mars bar** |

| | |
|---|---|
| 67 | Shredded wheat |
| 66 | Swiss museli |
| 66 | Brown rice |
| 64 | Raisins |
| 64 | Beets |
| 62 | Bananas |
| 59 | Sucrose |
| 59 | Sweet corn |
| 59 | Pastry |
| 51 | Bran |
| 51 | Green peas |
| 51 | Potato chips |
| 51 | Sweet potato |
| 50 | White spaghetti |
| 49 | Oatmeal |
| 45 | Grapes |
| 42 | Wholle grain rye bread |
| 42 | Whole wheat spaghetti |
| 40 | Orange |
| 39 | Apples |
| 38 | Tomatoes |
| 36 | Ice cream |
| 36 | Chick peas |
| 36 | Lima beans |
| 36 | Yogurt |
| 34 | Milk, whole |
| 32 | Milk, skim |
| 29 | Kidney beans |
| 29 | Lentils |
| 34 | Pears |
| 26 | Peaches |
| 26 | Grapefruiit |
| 25 | Plums |
| 23 | Cherries |
| 20 | Fructose |
| 15 | Soybeans |
| 13 | Peanuts |

# Index

# *Keats Good Herb Guides*

**Herbs for Improved Digestion** by CJ Puotinen
**Herbs to Help You Breathe Freely** by CJ Puotinen
**Herbs to Relieve Stress** by David Hoffmann
**Herbs to Relieve Arthritis** by CJ Puotinen
**Herbs for Headaches** by David Hoffmann
**Herbs for Womens' Health** by Mary Bove and Linda Costarella
**Herbs for Men's Health** by CJ Puotinen
**Herbs for The Heart** by CJ Putoinen
**Herbs for Detoxification** by CJ Putotinen
**Herbs for First Aid** by Penelope Ody
**Herbs for A Good Night's Sleep** by David Hoffmann
**Herbs to Boost Immunity** by Gail Ulrich
**Herbs to Relieve Chronic Fatigue** by Kathi Keville

**Gingko Biloba** by Frank Murray
**Ginseng** by Kathi Keville
**Echinacea** by Roy Upton
**Feverfew** by Ken Hancock
**Elder** by Brigitte Mars
**Kava Kava** by Robert Reichert
**St. John's Wort** by Roy Upton
**Calendula** by Mindy Green